Beautiful
MEMORY
Activities

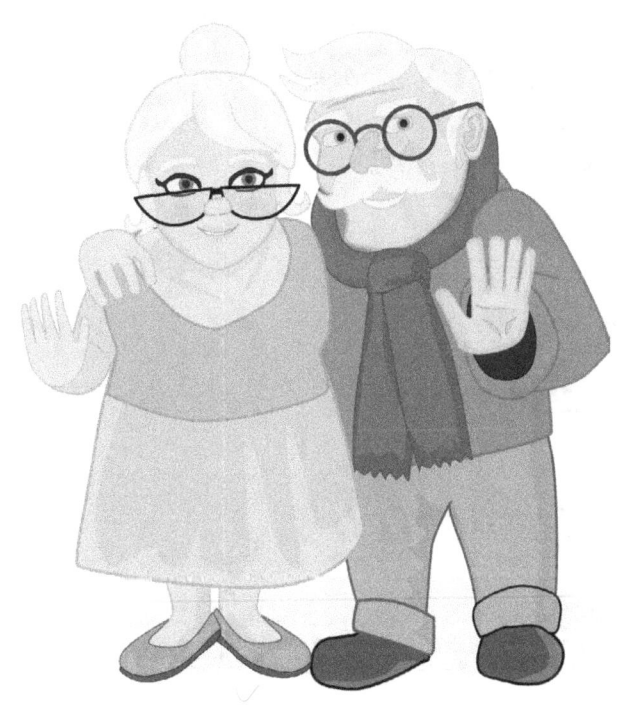

AUTUMN BOOKS

ISBN: 9798683205881

Images in this book are either in the public domain or from pixabay. com under the Pixabay License (2020), some of which have been adapted by Autumn Books.

Table of Contents

Introduction

Get ready to give your brain a full workout while having fun!

Short-term Memory

Remember new information for a short period to complete a task.

- **Flip the Page**: Memorize the contents of one page, then turn the page to complete a task.

- **Complete the Drawing**: A favorite of many, unleash your artistic side and use a grid to complete a simple drawing.

- **Memory Challenge!**: Remember a list of words, then turn the page and write as many words as you can.

Long-term Memory

Use information from the past.

- **Word Scramble**: Unscramble the themed words.

- **Categories**: Write as many words as you can in a given category.

- **Crosswords**: Clues are common sayings with missing words.

Working Memory and Classics

Improve focus and strengthen cognitive skills with classic puzzles like *Spot the Difference, Odd-One-Out, Find the Match,* and *Mazes.*

Spot the Difference

Find 5 differences between the 2 pictures on each page.

Spot the Difference 1

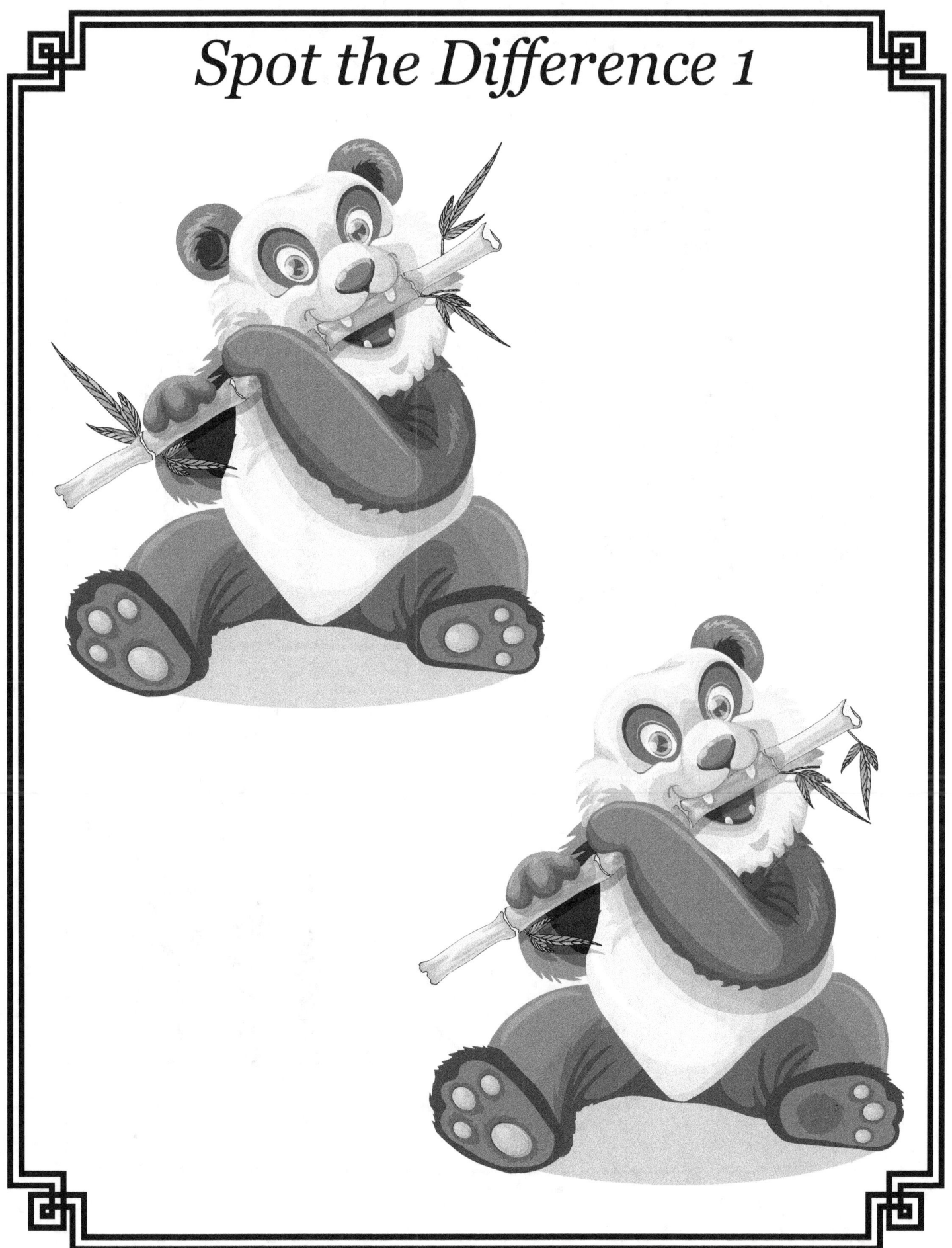

Spot the Difference 2

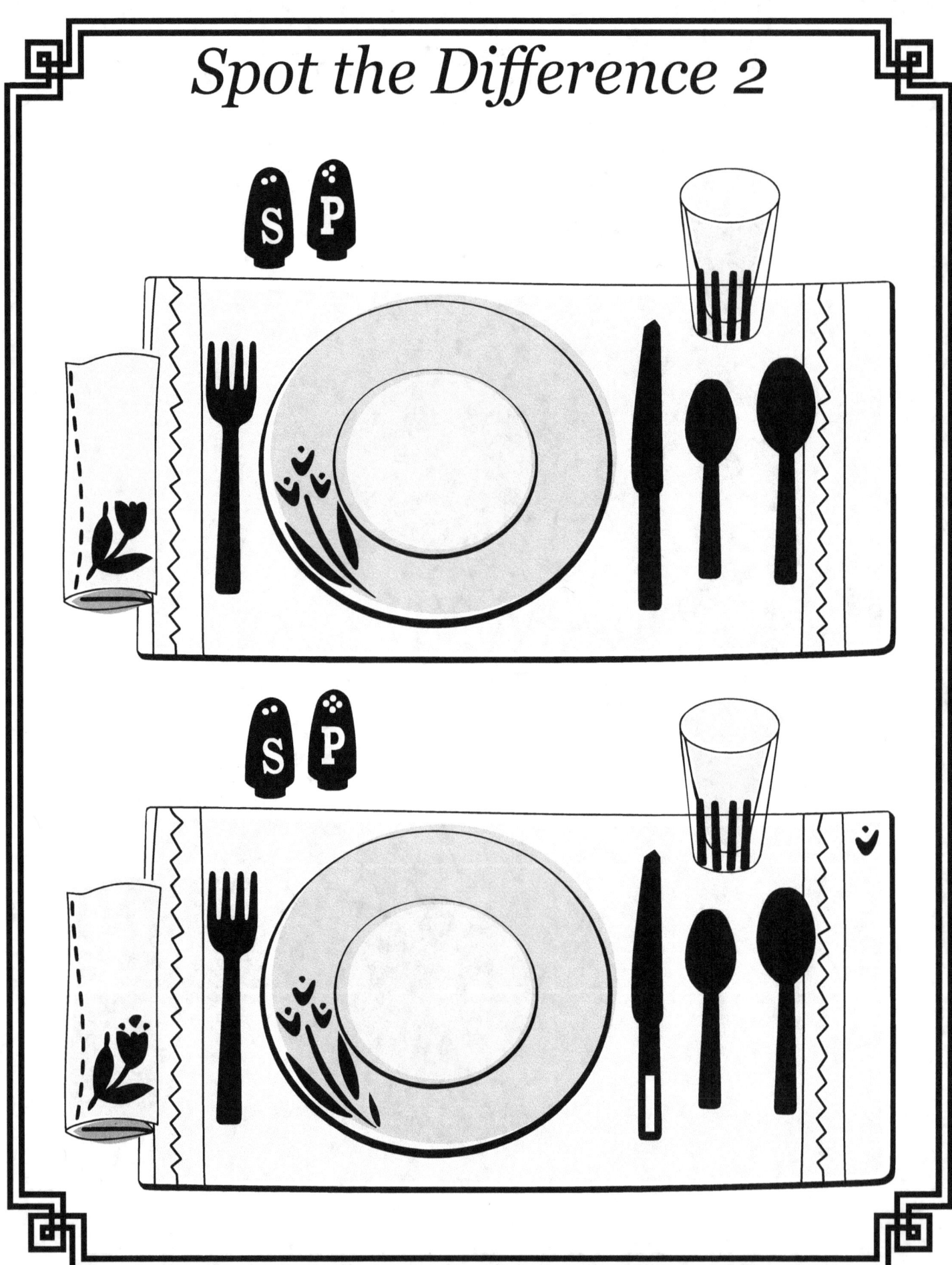

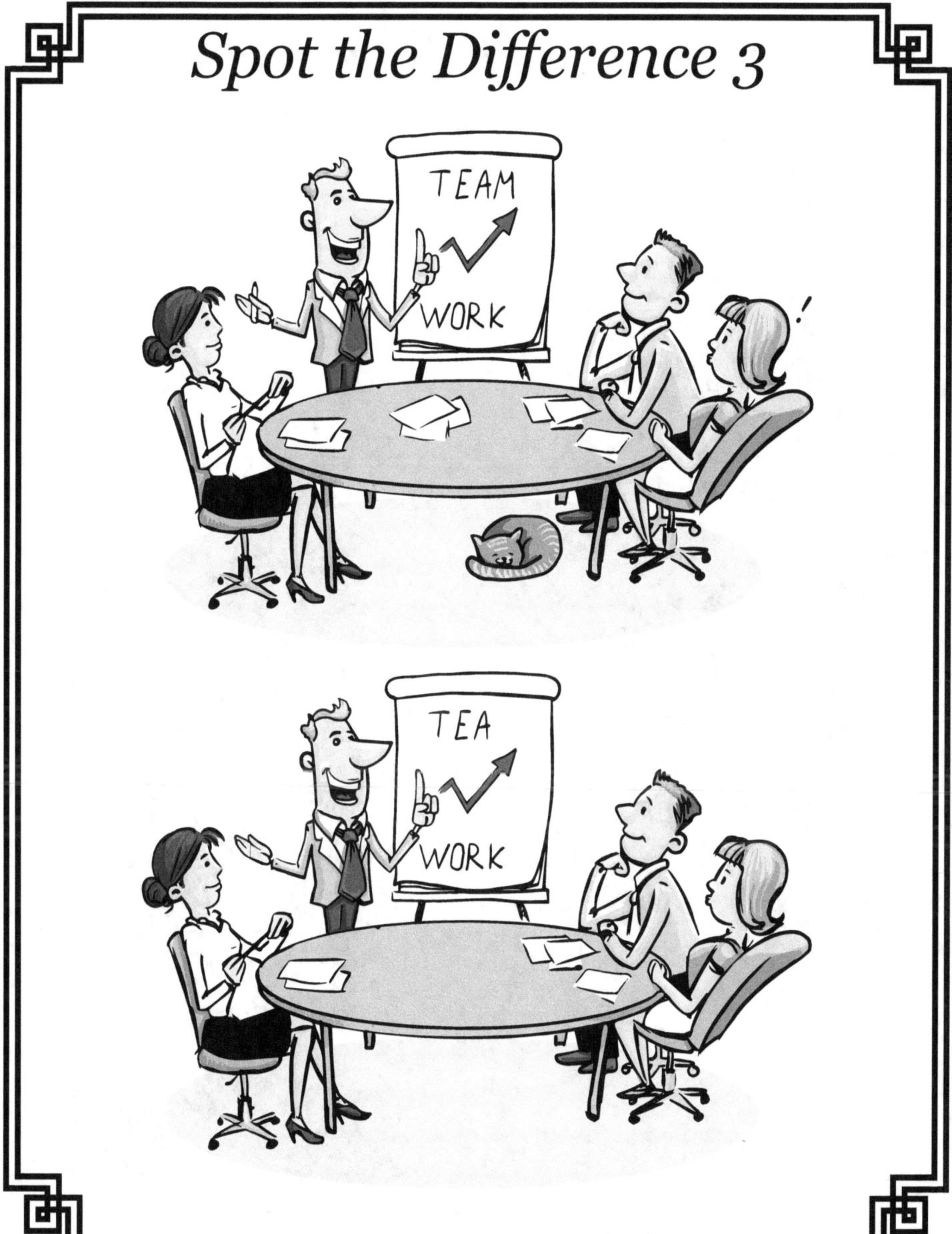

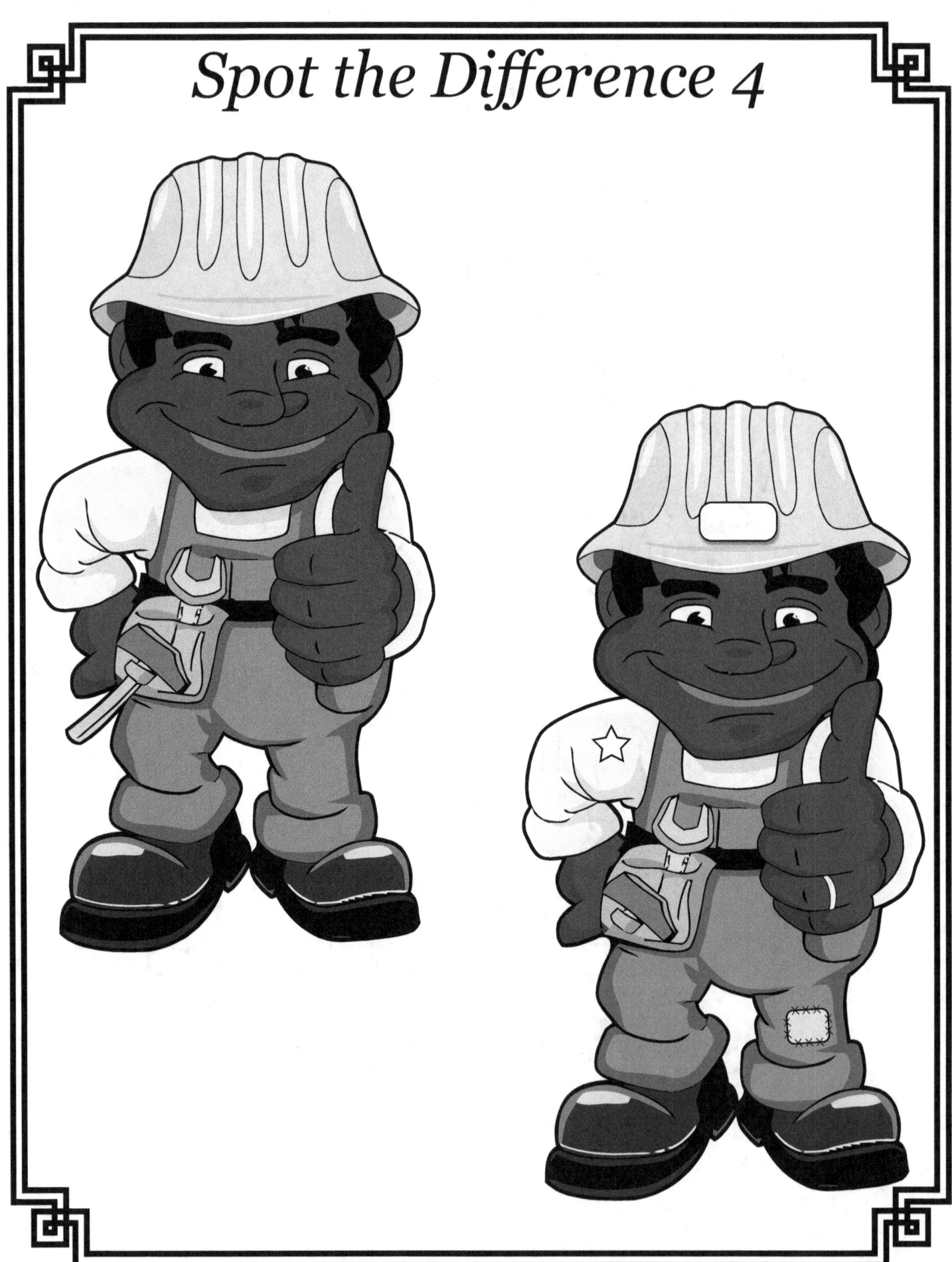

Spot the Difference 6

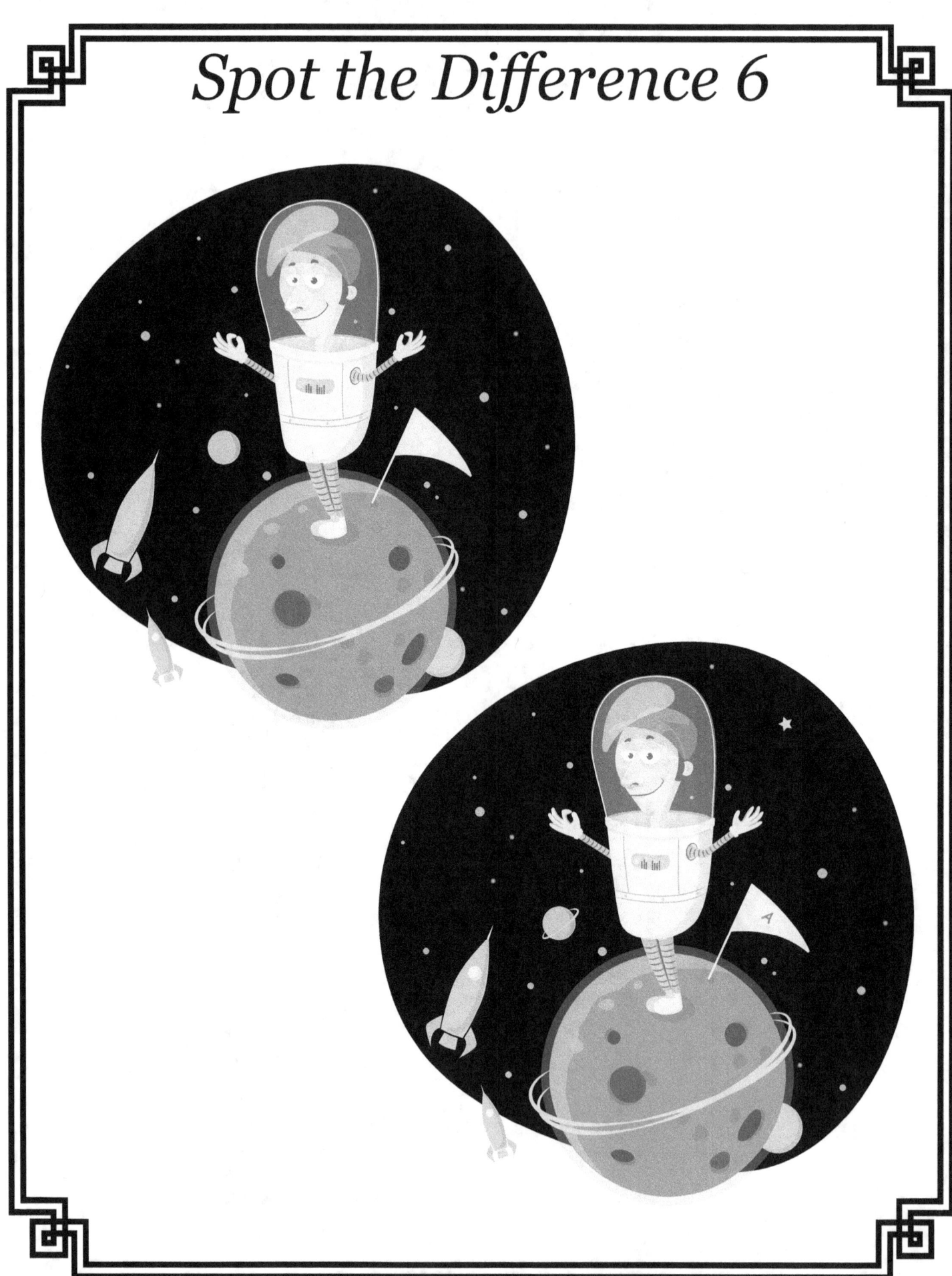

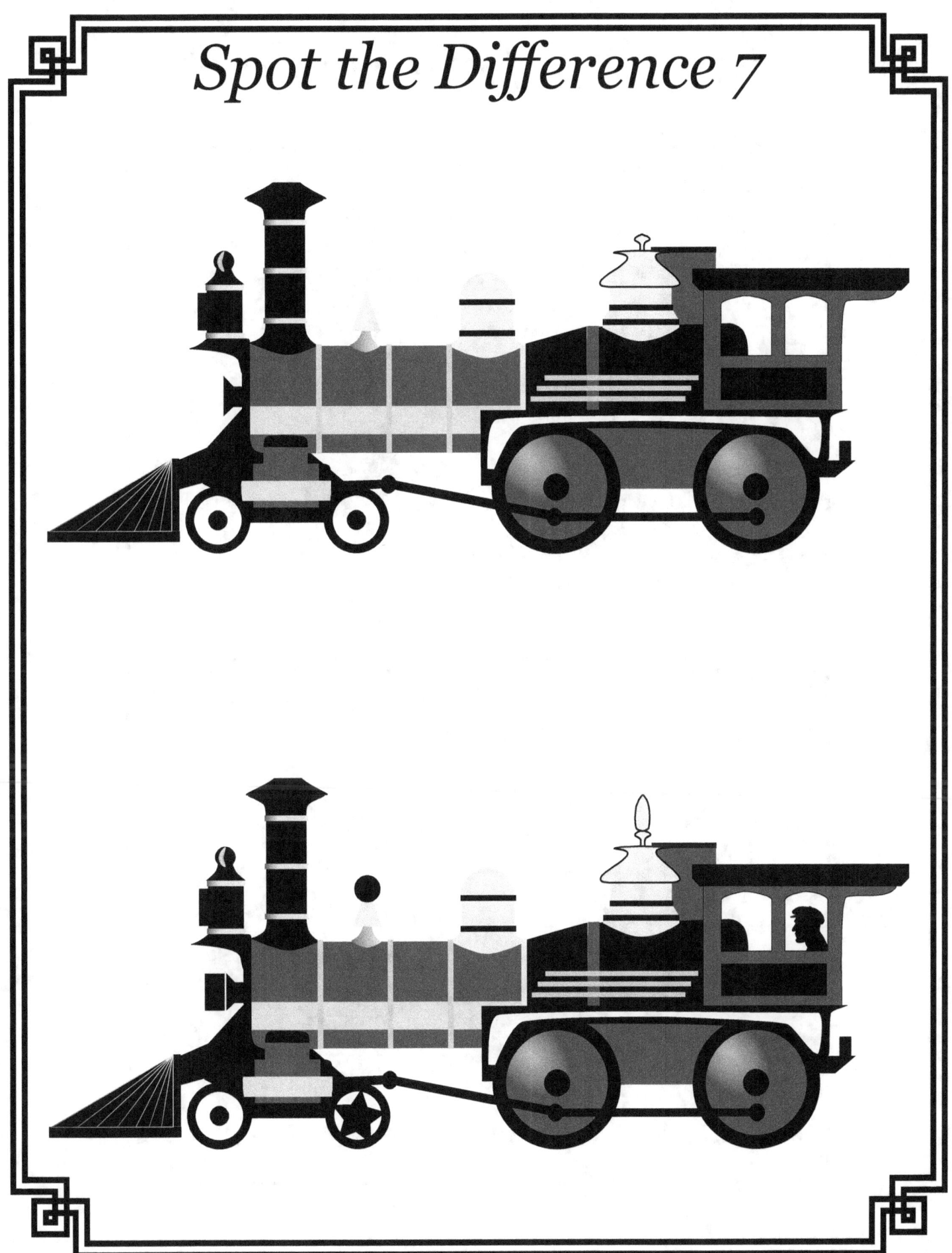

Spot the Difference 8

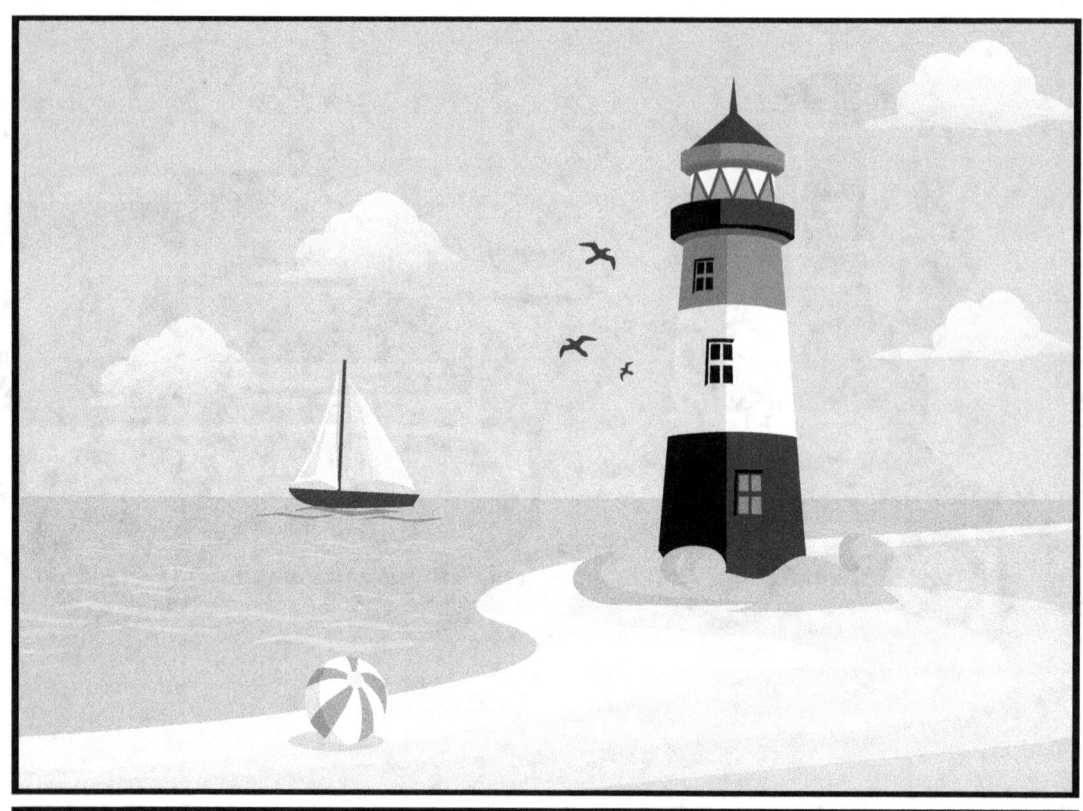

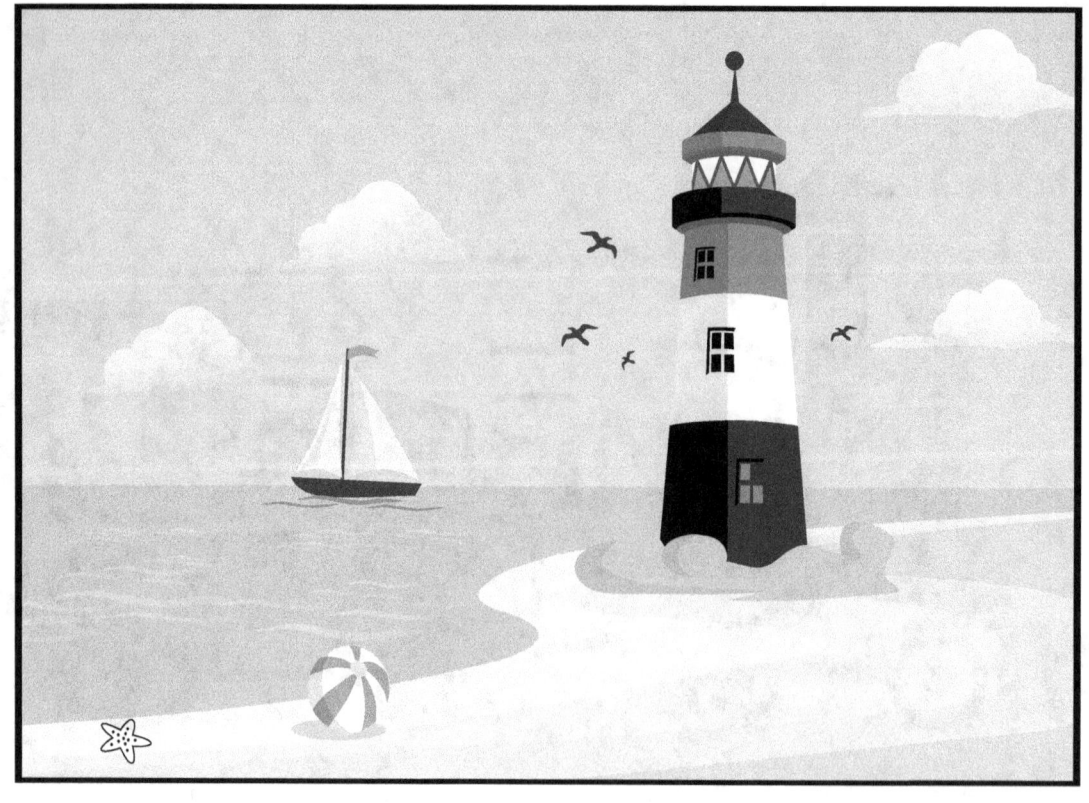

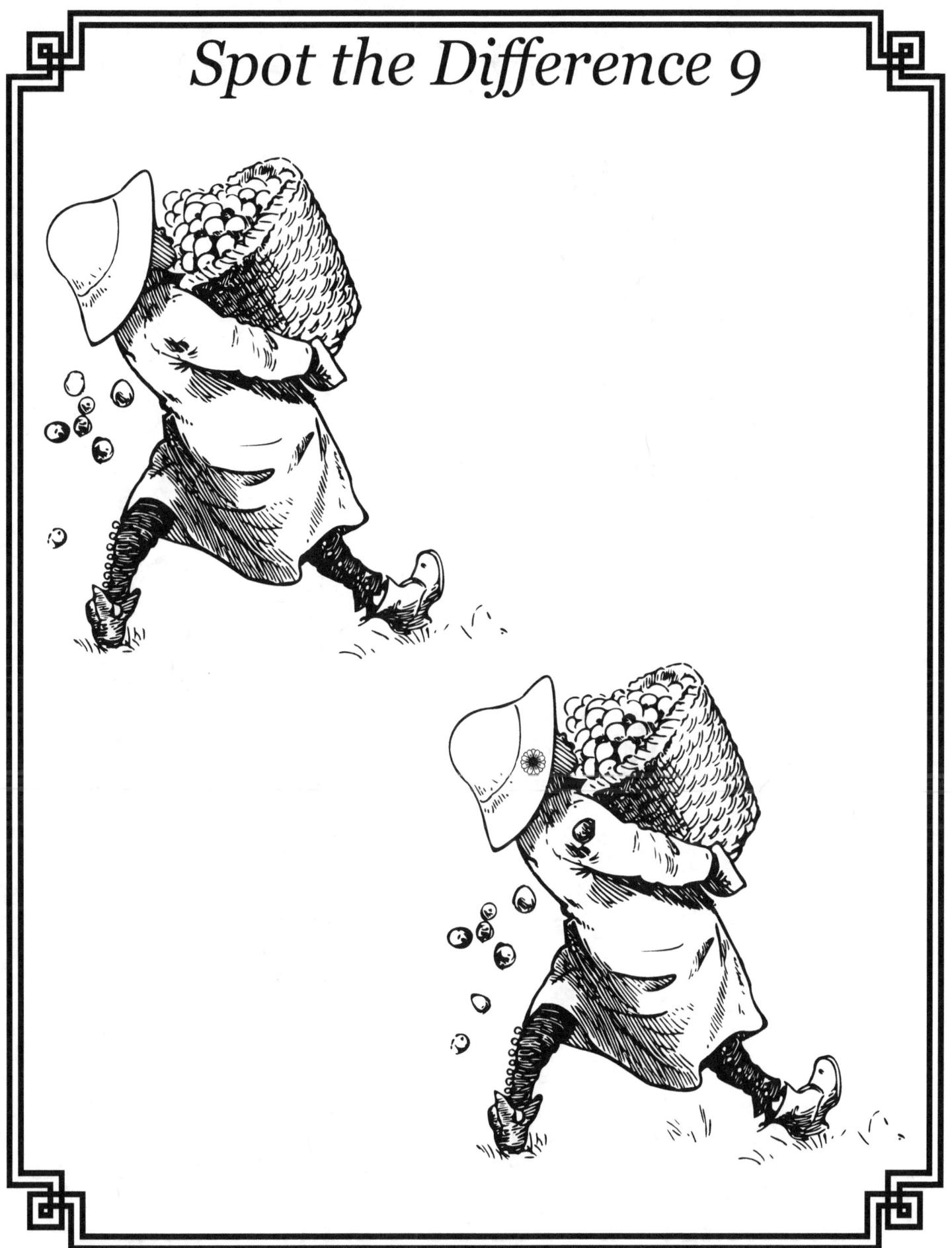

Spot the Difference 10

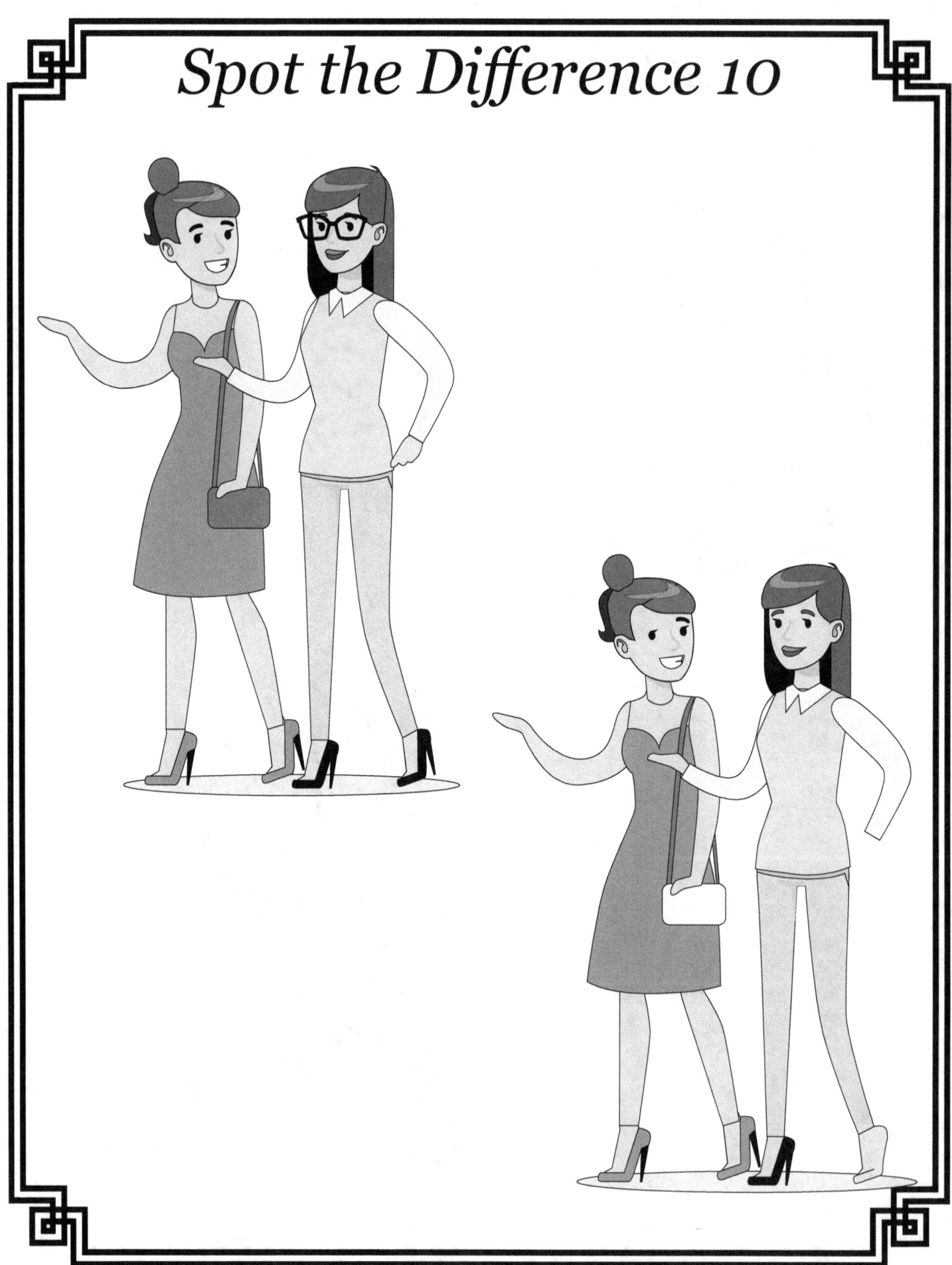

Spot the Difference Answers

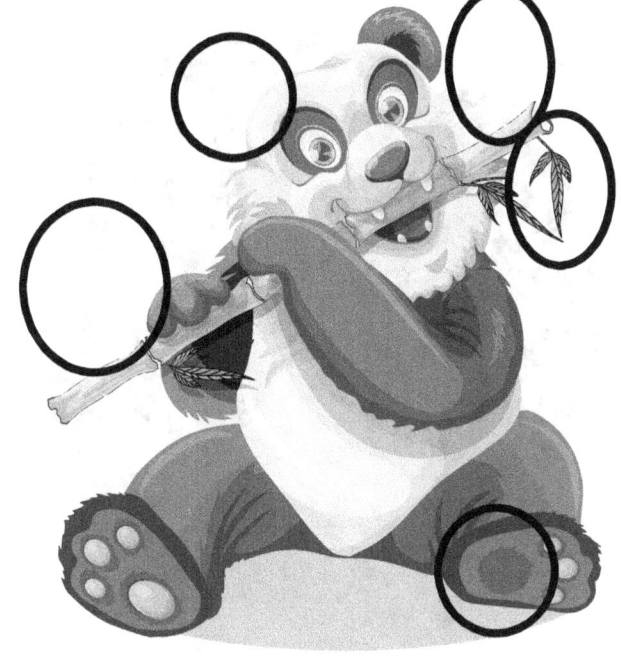

Spot the Difference 1

Spot the Difference 2

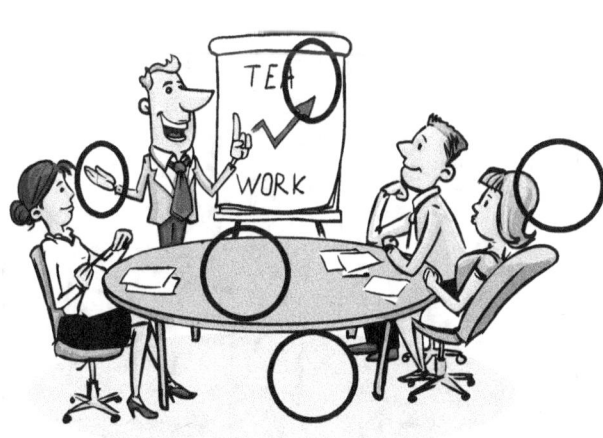

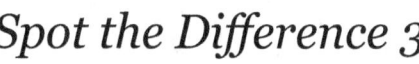

Spot the Difference 3

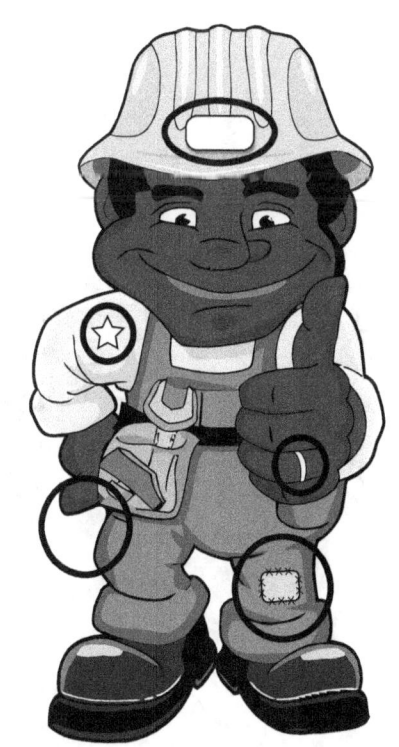

Spot the Difference 4

Spot the Difference Answers

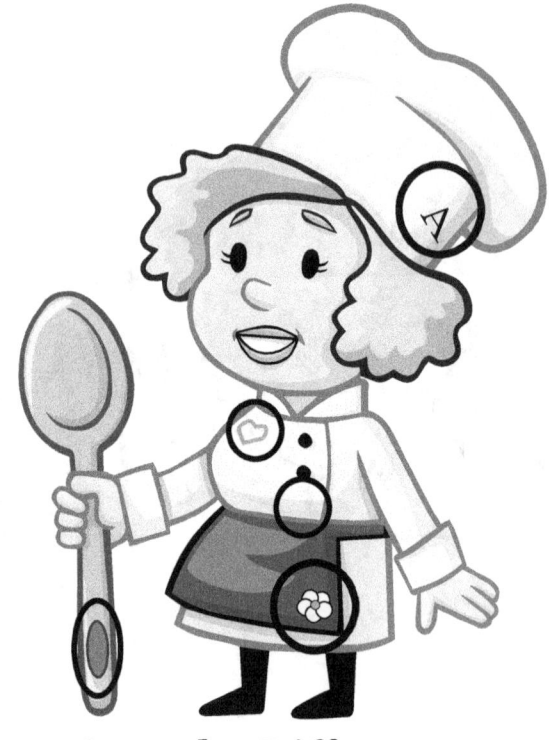

Spot the Difference 5

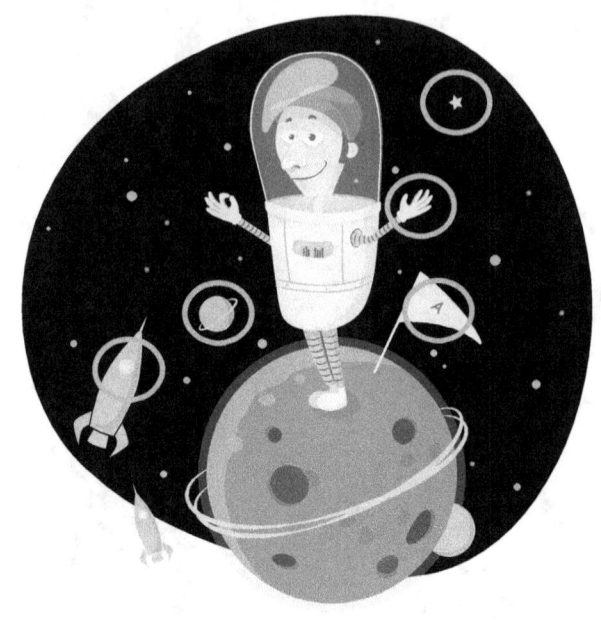

Spot the Difference 6

Spot the Difference 7

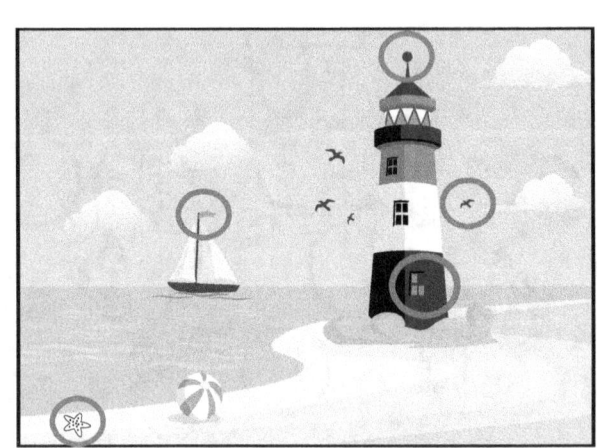

Spot the Difference 8

Spot the Difference Answers

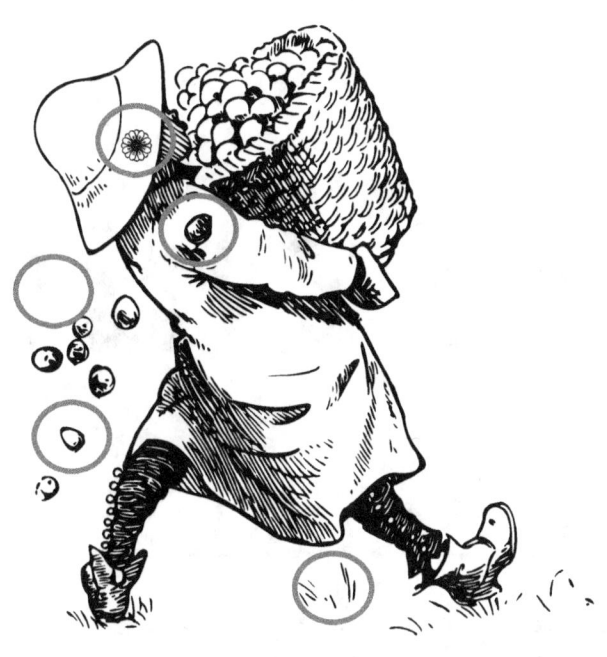

Spot the Difference 9

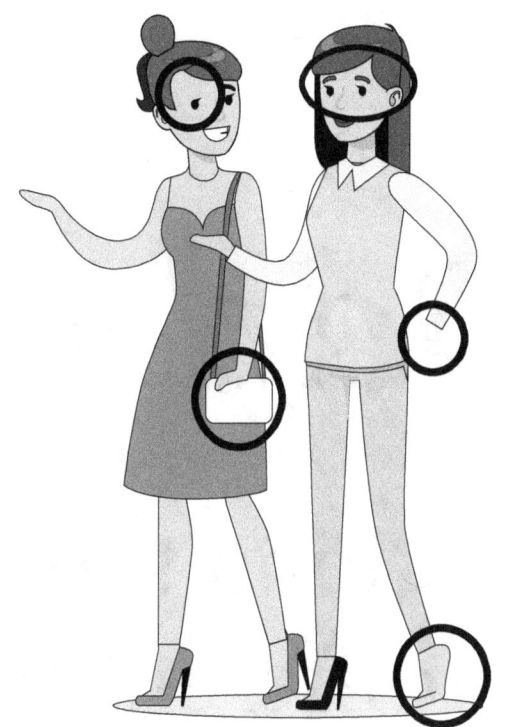

Spot the Difference 10

Odd-One-Out

Find the picture that is
different from the others.

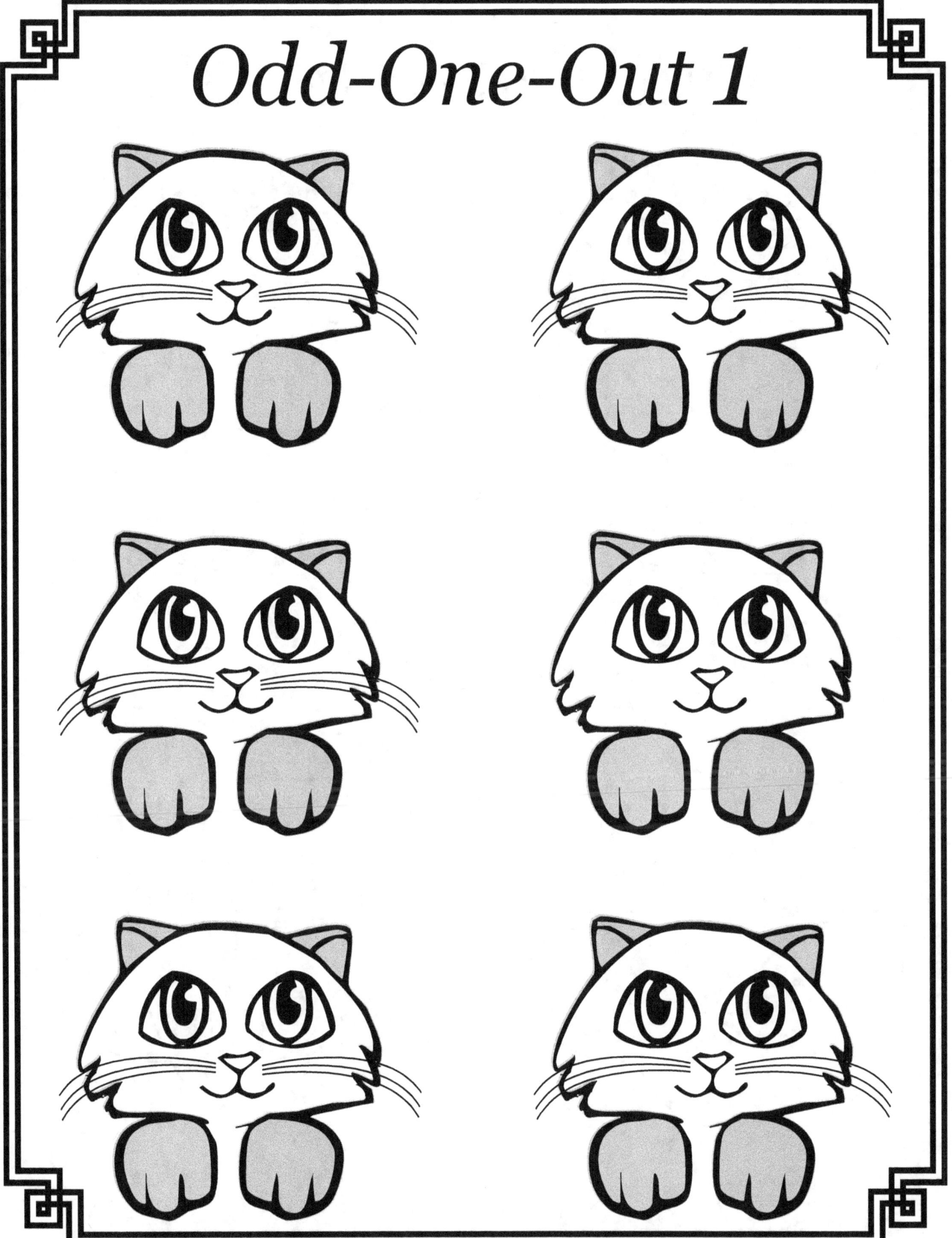

Odd-One-Out 2

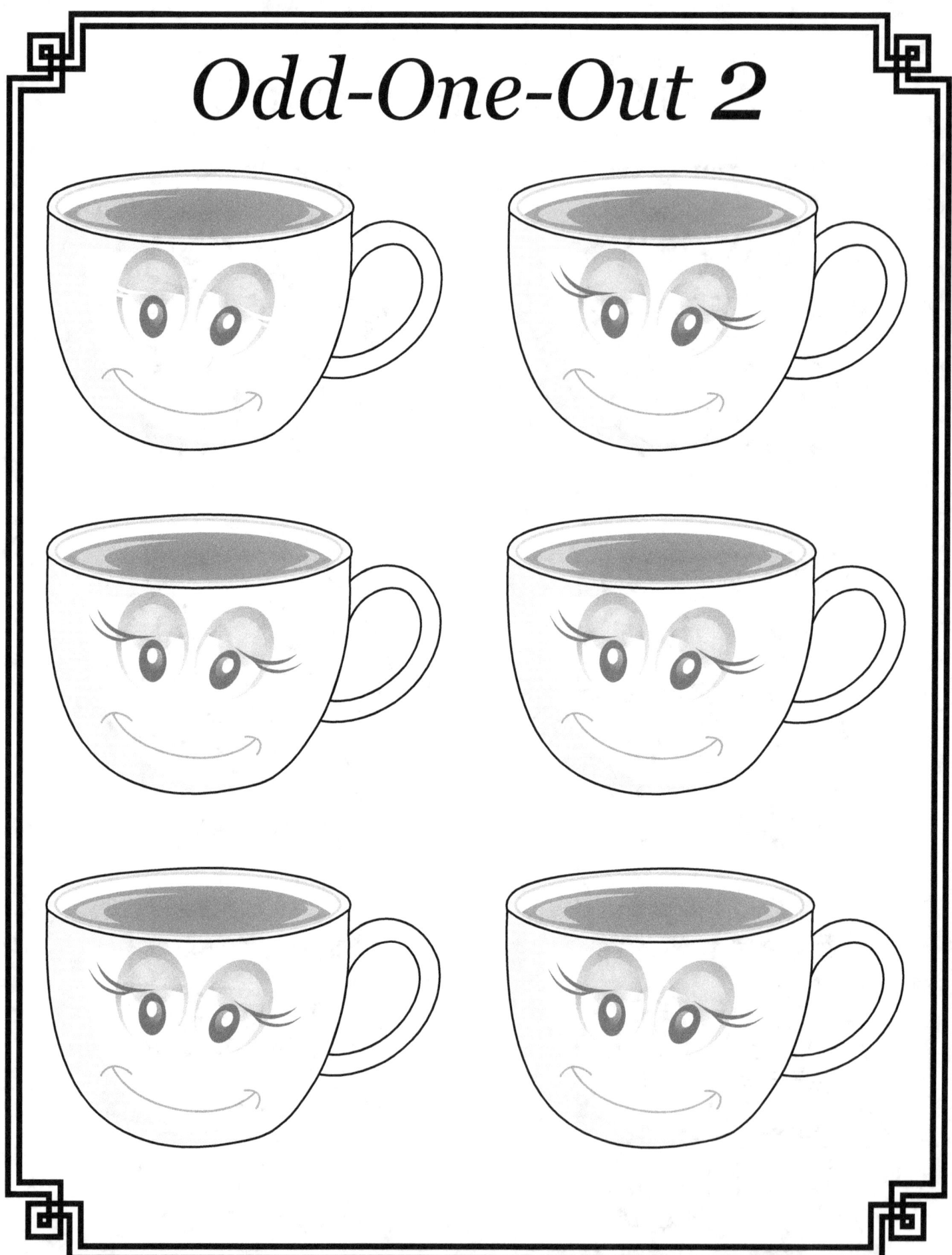

Odd-One-Out 3

Odd-One-Out 4

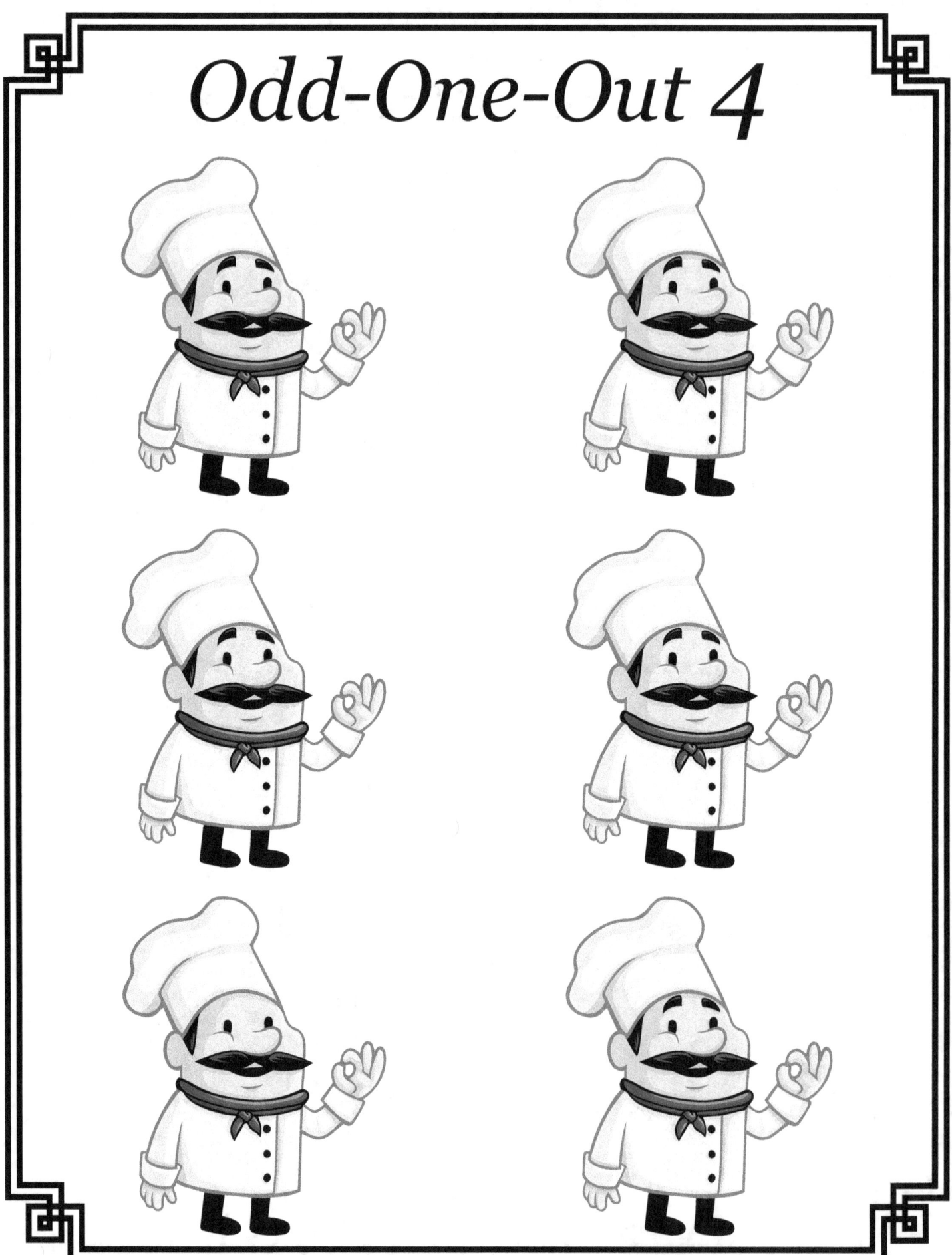

Odd-One-Out 5

Odd-One-Out 6

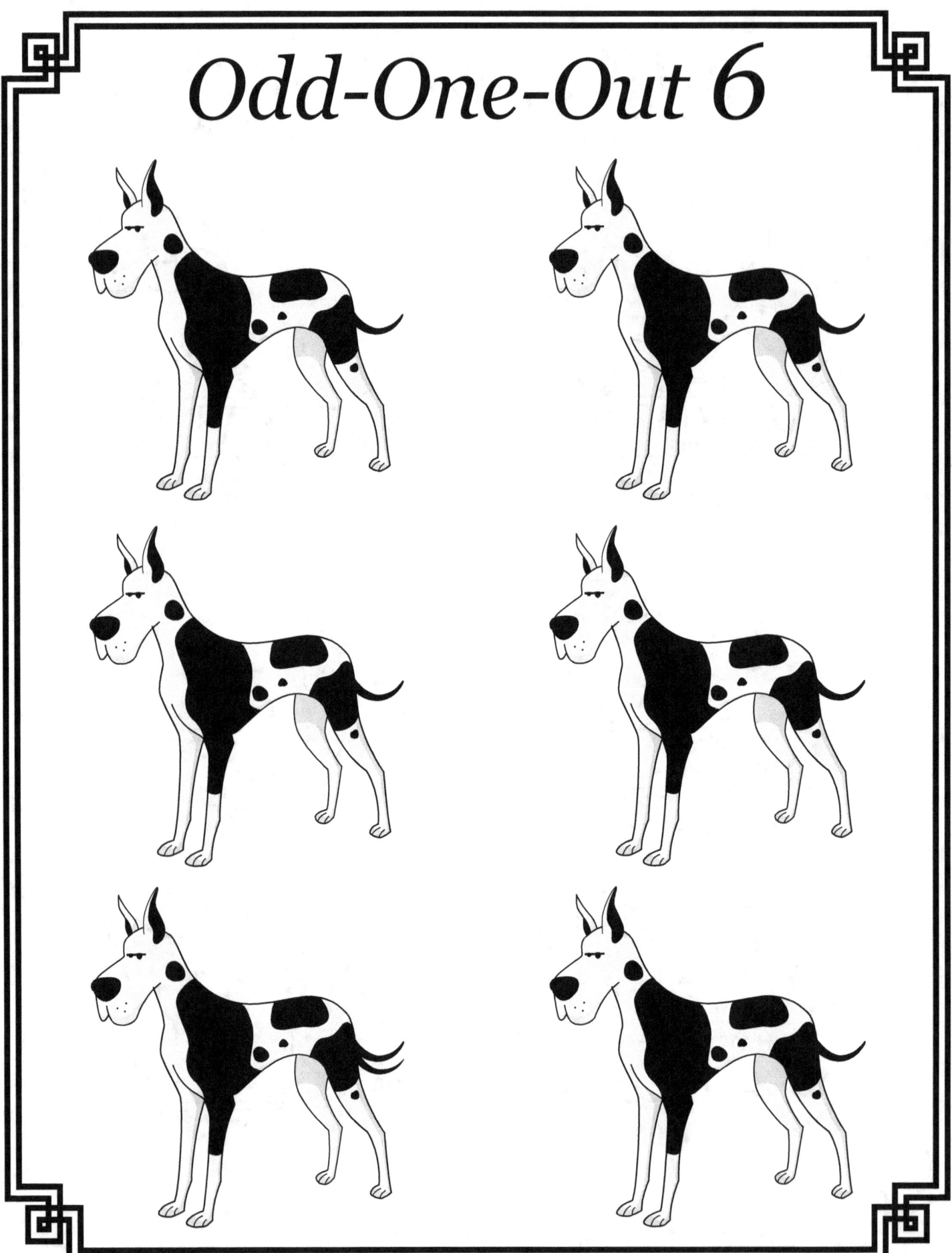

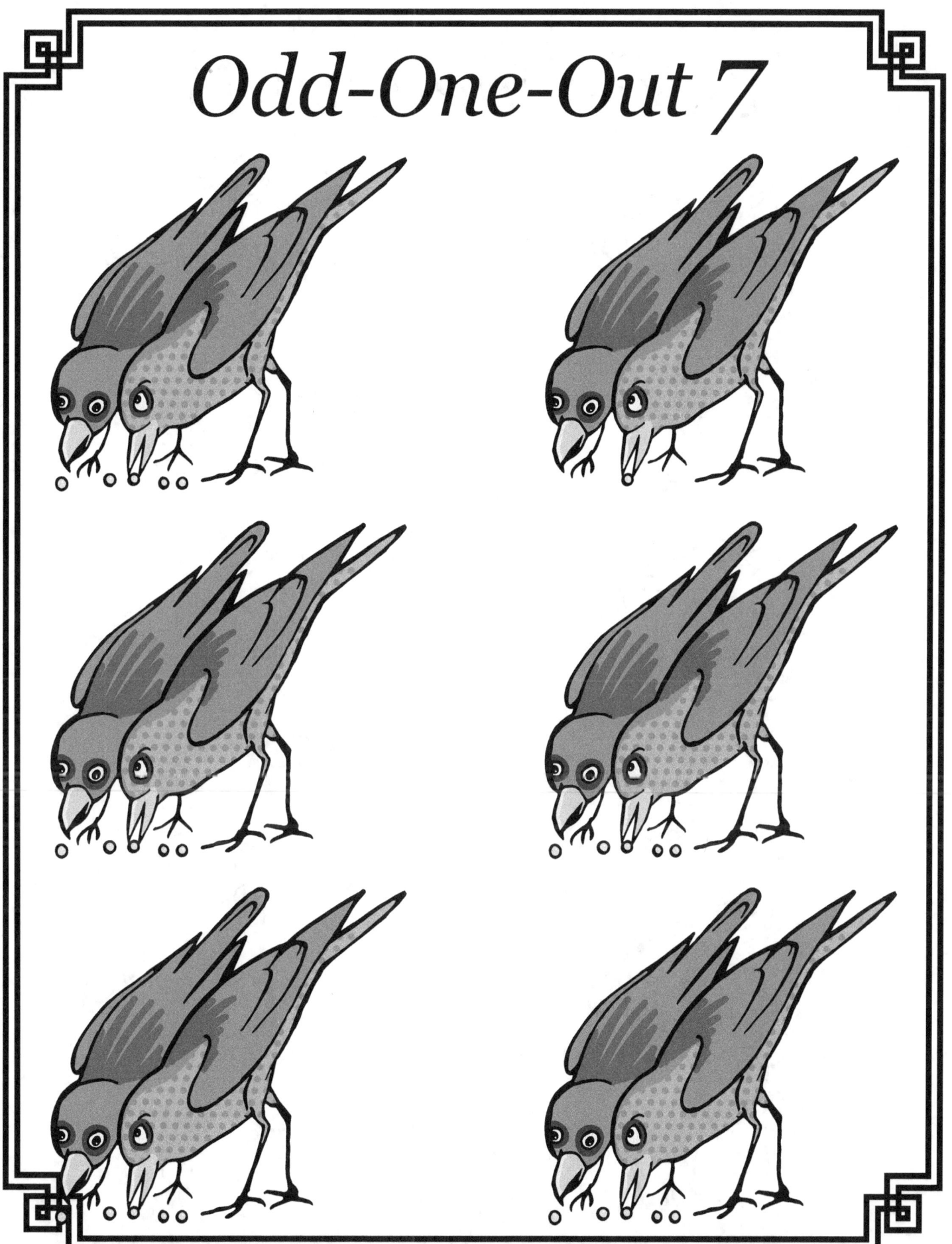

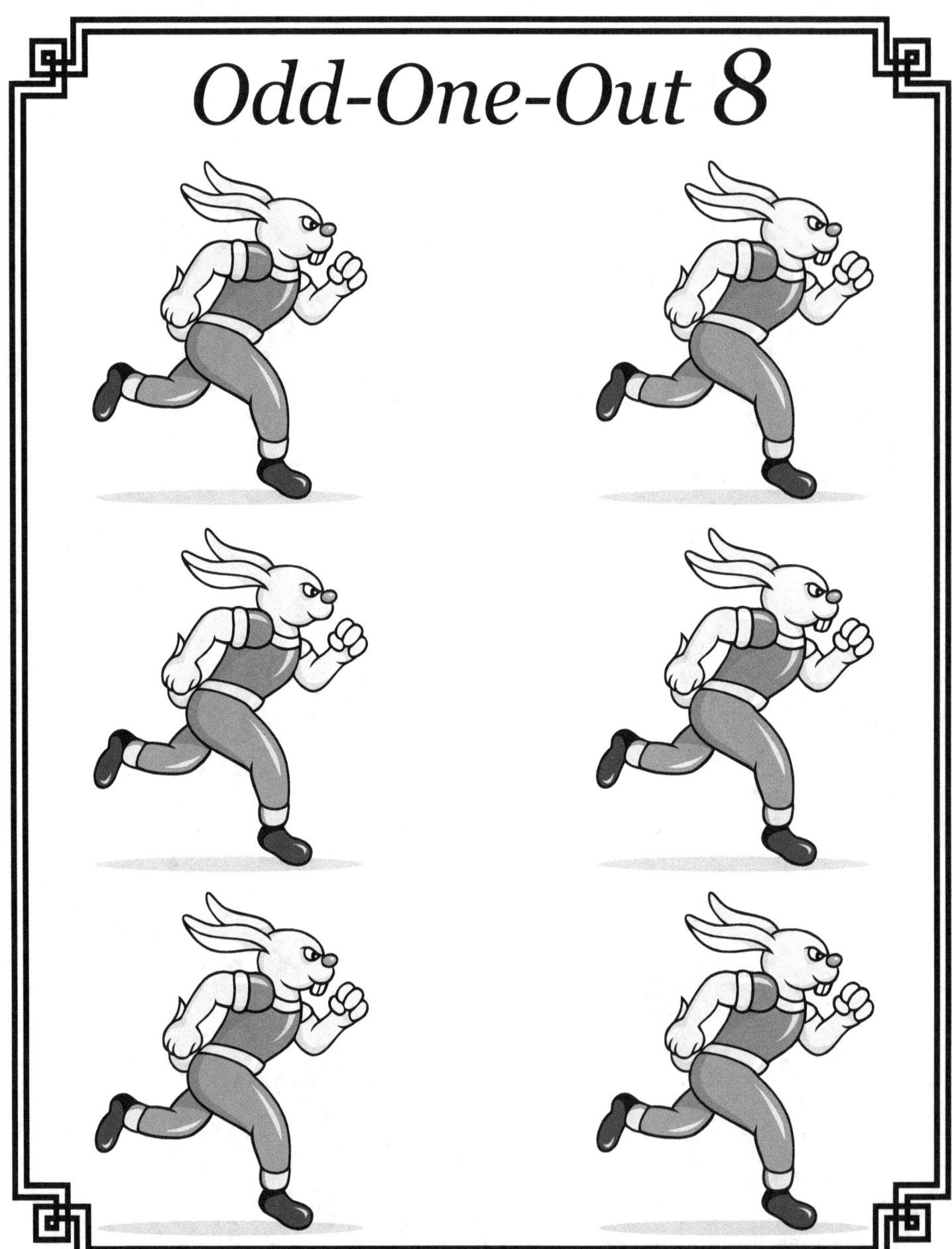

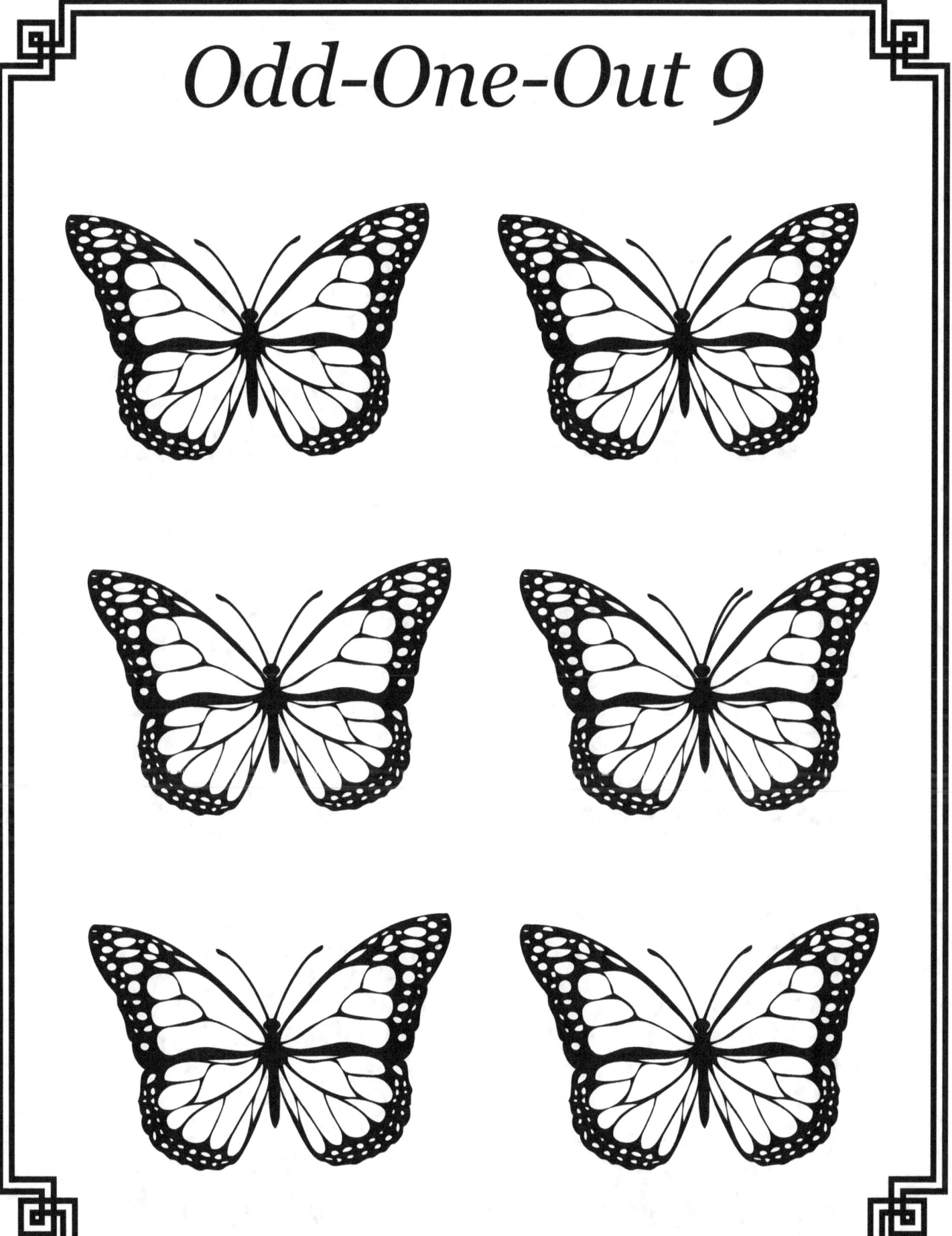

Odd-One-Out 10

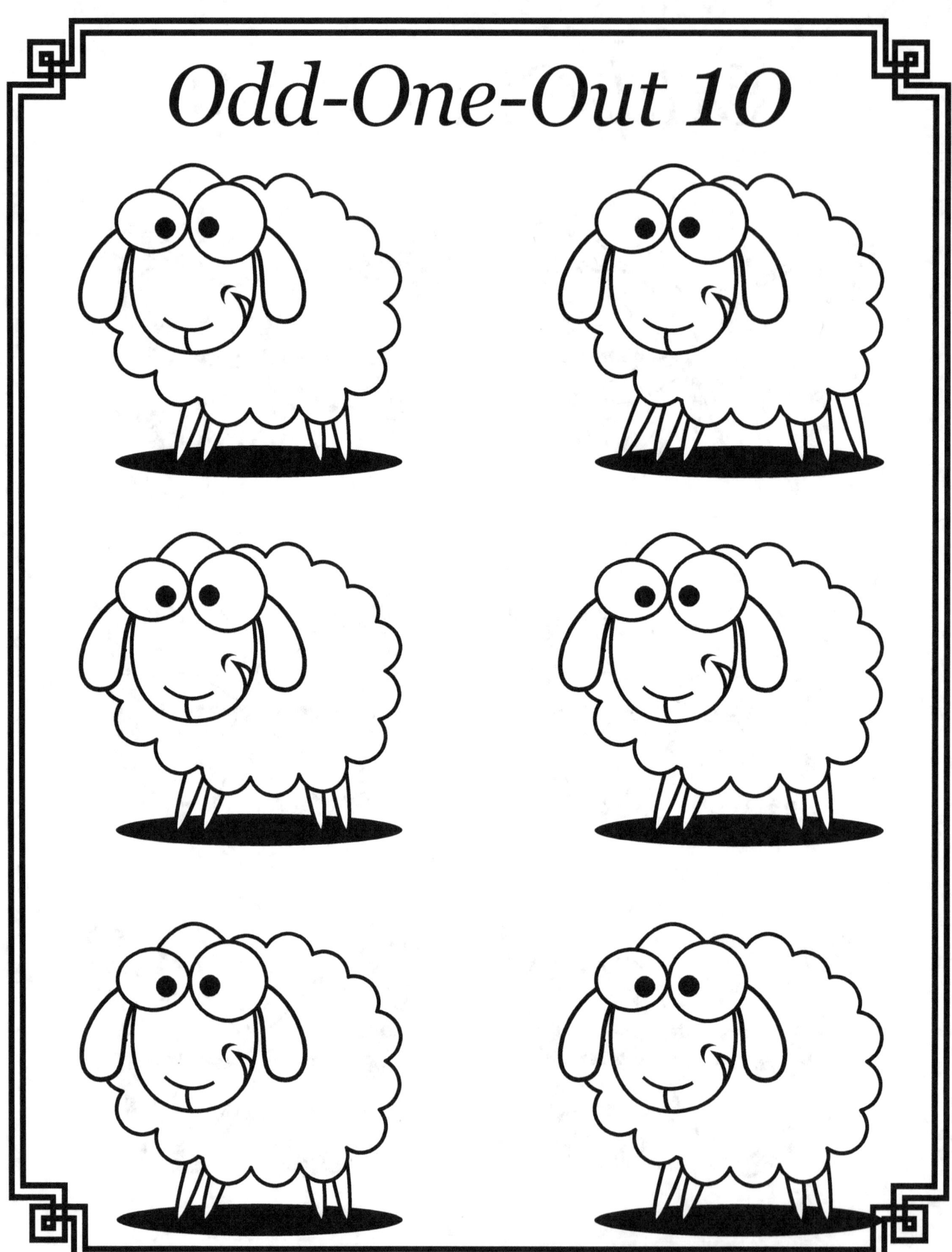

Odd-One-Out Answers

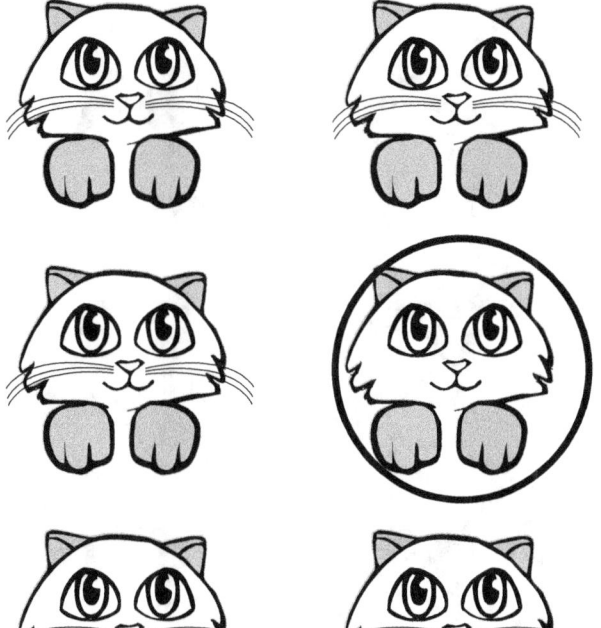

Odd-One-Out 1

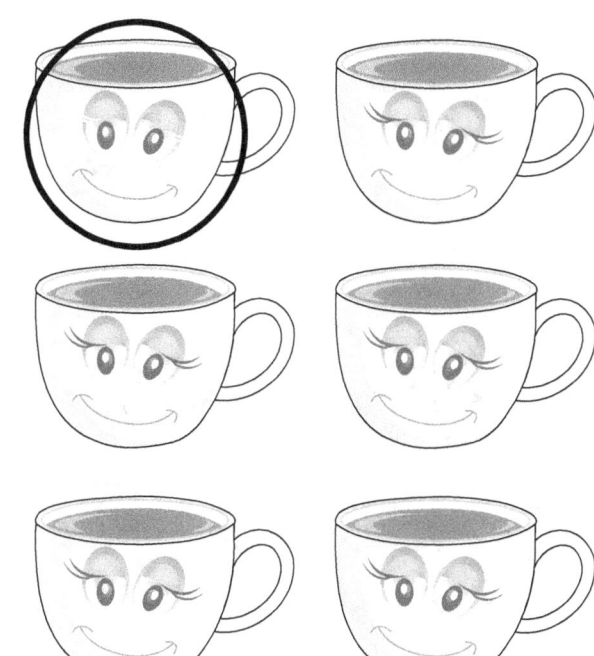

Odd-One-Out 2

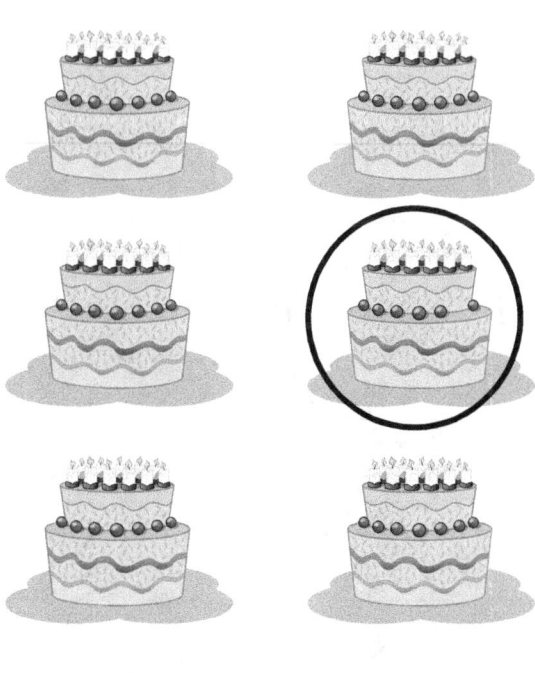

Odd-One-Out 3

Odd-One-Out 4

Odd-One-Out Answers

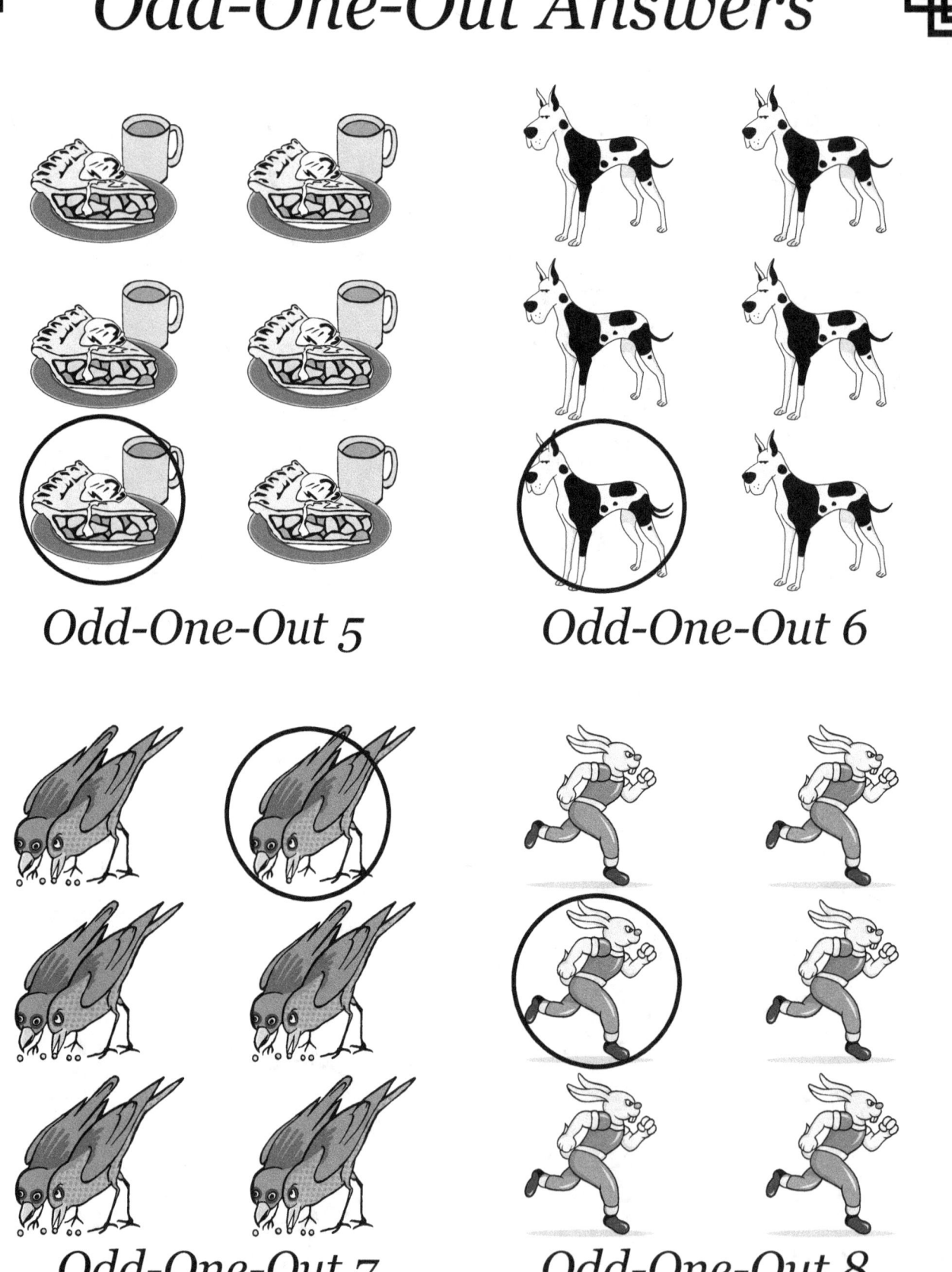

Odd-One-Out 5

Odd-One-Out 6

Odd-One-Out 7

Odd-One-Out 8

Odd-One-Out Answers

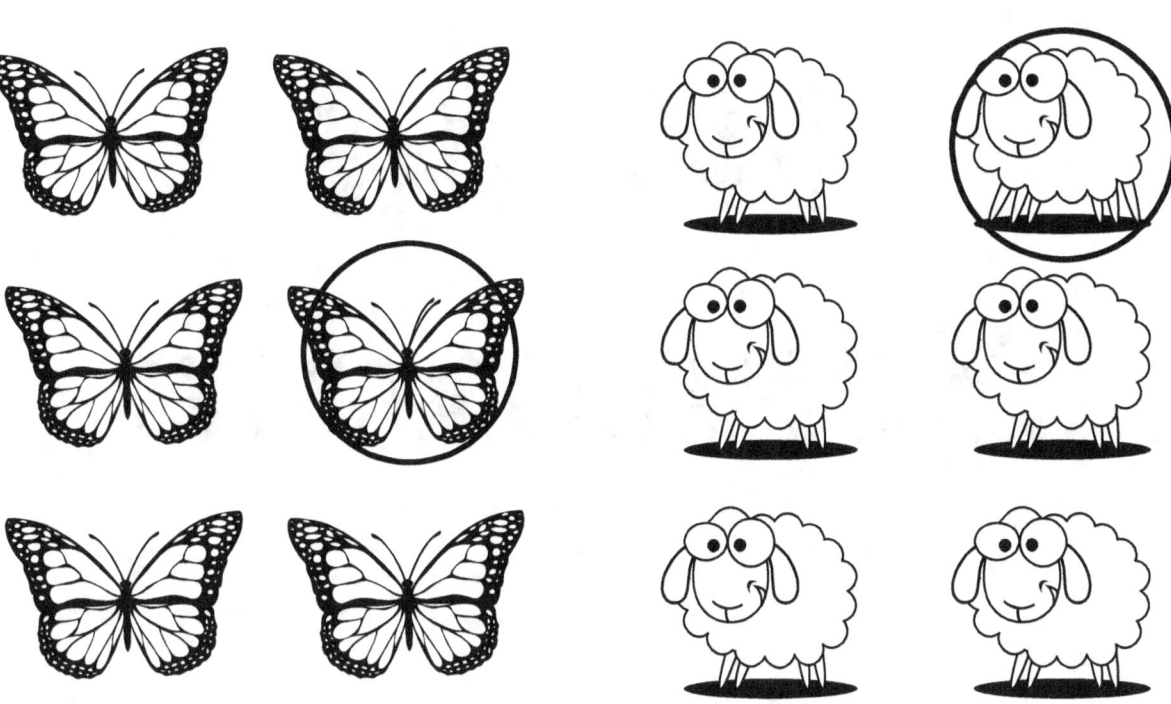

Odd-One-Out 9   *Odd-One-Out 10*

Word Scramble

Unscramble the words. Each word fits the theme at the top of the page.

Word Scramble 1
Tea Time

TAE   _____

CPU   _____

KMLI   _____

UARSG   _____

BISUCTI   _____

PORU   _____

POONS   _____

EETKTL   _____

Word Scramble 2
Weather

UYSNN   _____

ANIR   _____

NOSW   _____

OGF   _____

LCOD   _____

LUYCDO   _____

INDW   _____

TOH   _____

Word Scramble 3
Pets

TCA   _____

IHSF   _____

GDO   _____

DBRI   _____

KSEAN   _____

TARIBB   _____

TUETRL   _____

RTHAESM   _____

Word Scramble 4
Instruments

ABTU   _____

ABSS   _____

RHAP   _____

OINAP   _____

MDRU   _____

GANOR   _____

UFTLE   _____

IUATRG   _____

Breakfast

GGES   _____

CEFEOF   _____

AEAKCPN   _____

PRUYS   _____

CANBO   _____

FFLWEA   _____

AECLRE   _____

SAEUGAS   _____

Word Scramble Answers

TEA	SUNNY
CUP	RAIN
MILK	SNOW
SUGAR	FOG
BISCUIT	COLD
POUR	CLOUDY
SPOON	WIND
KETTLE	HOT
Word Scramble 1	Word Scramble 2
CAT	TUBA
FISH	BASS
DOG	HARP
BIRD	PIANO
SNAKE	DRUM
RABBIT	ORGAN
TURTLE	FLUTE
HAMSTER	GUITAR
Word Scramble 3	Word Scramble 4

Word Scramble Answers

EGGS

COFFEE

PANCAKE

SYRUP

BACON

WAFFLE

CEREAL

SAUSAGE

Word Scramble 5

Flip the Page

Part 1: Memorize the sentence on the page, then flip the page and select the same sentence from the choices.

Part 2: Memorize the list of words, then flip the page and select the same words from the grid of related words.

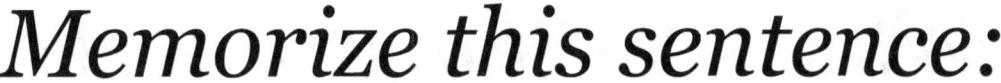

Memorize this sentence:

Jane walked to the store on Sunday to buy milk.

Which sentence was it?

A Jane walked to the store on Sunday to buy mayo.

B Jane walked to the store on Saturday to buy milk.

C Jane walked to the store on Sunday to buy milk.

D Joan walked to the store on Sunday to buy mayo.

Flip back to check your answer.

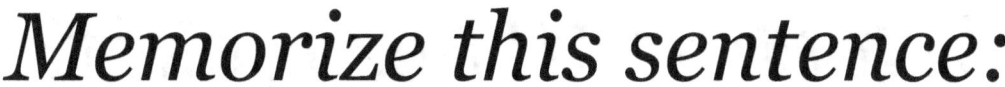

Memorize this sentence:

The brown dog fetched the stick at Howard Park.

Which sentence was it?

A The dark brown dog fetched the stick at Howard Way.

B The brown dog fetched the twig at the Howard Way.

C The brown dog fetched the stick at the Hyatt Park.

D The brown dog fetched the stick at the Howard Park.

Flip back to check your answer.

Memorize this sentence:

The birthday party last week was fantastic, wasn't it?

Which sentence was it?

A The birthday party last week was fantastic, wasn't it?

B The birthday cake last week was fantastic, wasn't it?

C The birthday cake this week was fantastic, wasn't it?

D The birthday party this week was fantastic, right?

Flip back to check your answer.

Memorize this sentence:

I hope the Wildcats beat the Lions in the basketball game tomorrow night.

Which sentence was it?

A I hope the Lions beat the Wildcats in the baseball game tomorrow night.

B I hope the Wildcats beat the Lions in the baseball game tomorrow night.

C I hope the Wildcats beat the Lions in the basketball game tomorrow night.

D I hope the Wildcats beat the Lions in the basketball game tonight.

Flip back to check your answer.

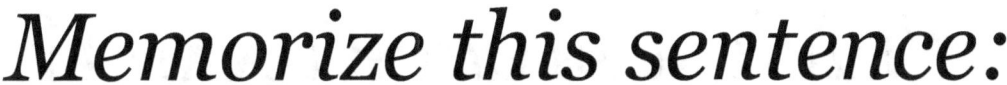

Memorize this sentence:

Those roses in Mary and Jim's garden came in so well!

Which sentence was it?

A Those roses in Jim and Mary's garden came in great!

B Those roses in Mary and Jim's garden came in so well!

C The roses in Jim and Mary's garden came in so well!

D Those daisies in Mary and Jim's garden came in so well!

Flip back to check your answer.

Memorize this list of words:

EGGS

BUTTER

MILK

WAFFLES

JUICE

COFFEE

Which words were on the previous page?

COFFEE	CEREAL	BACON
BUTTER	EGGS	WAFFLES
MILK	JUICE	SAUSAGE

Flip back to check your answer.

Memorize this list of words:

ROSE

DAISY

LILY

DAHLIA

PEONY

LILAC

Which words were on the previous page?

LAVENDER	DAISY	PEONY
LILY	TULIP	ROSE
LILAC	DAHILA	PANSY

Flip back to check your answer.

Memorize this list of words:

HAMMER

WRENCH

PLIERS

SCREW

NAIL

SANDER

Which words were on the previous page?

SCREW	NUT	HAMMER
PLIERS	WRENCH	SAW
NAIL	SANDER	RULER

Flip back to check your answer.

Memorize this list of words:

CLOUD

SUN

WIND

RAIN

SNOW

SLEET

HOT

CHILL

Which words were on the previous page?

SNOW	CLOUD	HEAT
COLD	CHILL	SUN
HOT	HUMID	SLEET
RAIN	SUNNY	WIND

Flip back to check your answer.

Memorize this list of words:

BAKER

BUTCHER

FIREMAN

DOCTOR

NURSE

TEACHER

LAWYER

ARTIST

Which words were on the previous page?

POLICEMAN	BAKER	ARTIST
FIREMAN	CHEF	LAWYER
DOCTOR	BUTCHER	JUDGE
PLUMMER	NURSE	TEACHER

Flip back to check your answer.

Categories

Write as many words as possible in the category at the top of each page.

Added challenge: Set a timer for 2 minutes

Cooking

1. _____
2. _____
3. _____
4. _____
5. _____
6. _____
7. _____
8. _____
9. _____
10. _____
11. _____
12. _____
13. _____
14. _____
15. _____
16. _____
16. _____
17. _____
19. _____
19. _____
20. _____
20. _____
21. _____
22. _____
23. _____
24. _____
25. _____
26. _____
27. _____
28. _____
29. _____
30. _____
31. _____
32. _____
33. _____
34. _____
35. _____
36. _____
37. _____
38. _____
39. _____
40. _____
41. _____
42. _____
43. _____
44. _____
45. _____
46. _____
47. _____
48. _____
49. _____
50. _____
51. _____
52. _____

Sports

1. _____
2. _____
3. _____
4. _____
5. _____
6. _____
7. _____
8. _____
9. _____
10. _____
11. _____
12. _____
13. _____
14. _____
15. _____
16. _____
16. _____
17. _____
19. _____
19. _____
20. _____
20. _____
21. _____
22. _____
23. _____
24. _____
25. _____
26. _____
27. _____
28. _____
29. _____
30. _____
31. _____
32. _____
33. _____
34. _____
35. _____
36. _____
37. _____
38. _____
39. _____
40. _____
41. _____
42. _____
43. _____
44. _____
45. _____
46. _____
47. _____
48. _____
49. _____
50. _____
51. _____
52. _____

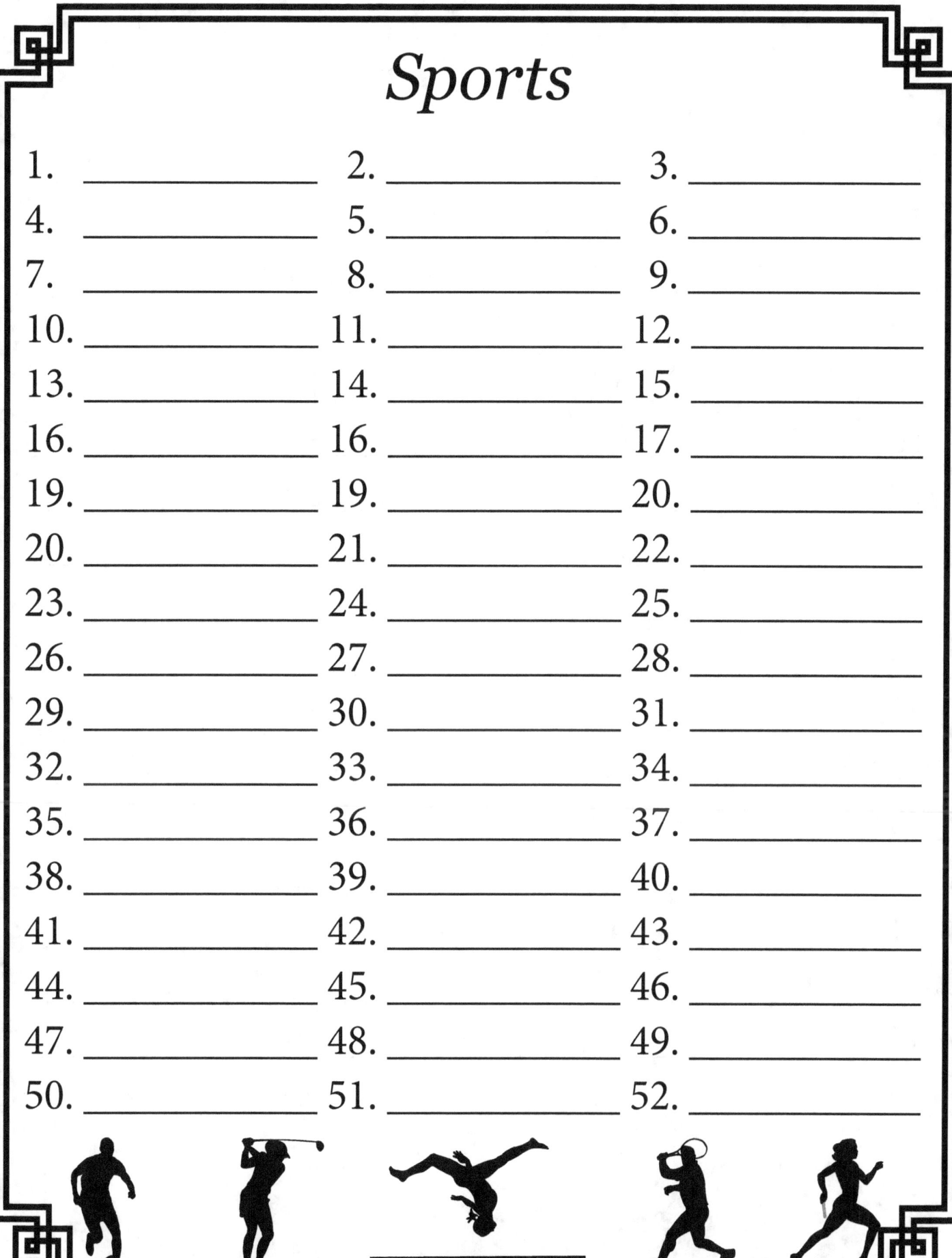

Summer

1. _____ 2. _____ 3. _____

4. _____ 5. _____ 6. _____

7. _____ 8. _____ 9. _____

10. _____ 11. _____ 12. _____

13. _____ 14. _____ 15. _____

16. _____ 16. _____ 17. _____

19. _____ 19. _____ 20. _____

20. _____ 21. _____ 22. _____

23. _____ 24. _____ 25. _____

26. _____ 27. _____ 28. _____

29. _____ 30. _____ 31. _____

32. _____ 33. _____ 34. _____

35. _____ 36. _____ 37. _____

38. _____ 39. _____ 40. _____

41. _____ 42. _____ 43. _____

44. _____ 45. _____ 46. _____

47. _____ 48. _____ 49. _____

50. _____ 51. _____ 52. _____

Jobs

1. _____
2. _____
3. _____
4. _____
5. _____
6. _____
7. _____
8. _____
9. _____
10. _____
11. _____
12. _____
13. _____
14. _____
15. _____
16. _____
16. _____
17. _____
19. _____
19. _____
20. _____
20. _____
21. _____
22. _____
23. _____
24. _____
25. _____
26. _____
27. _____
28. _____
29. _____
30. _____
31. _____
32. _____
33. _____
34. _____
35. _____
36. _____
37. _____
38. _____
39. _____
40. _____
41. _____
42. _____
43. _____
44. _____
45. _____
46. _____
47. _____
48. _____
49. _____
50. _____
51. _____
52. _____

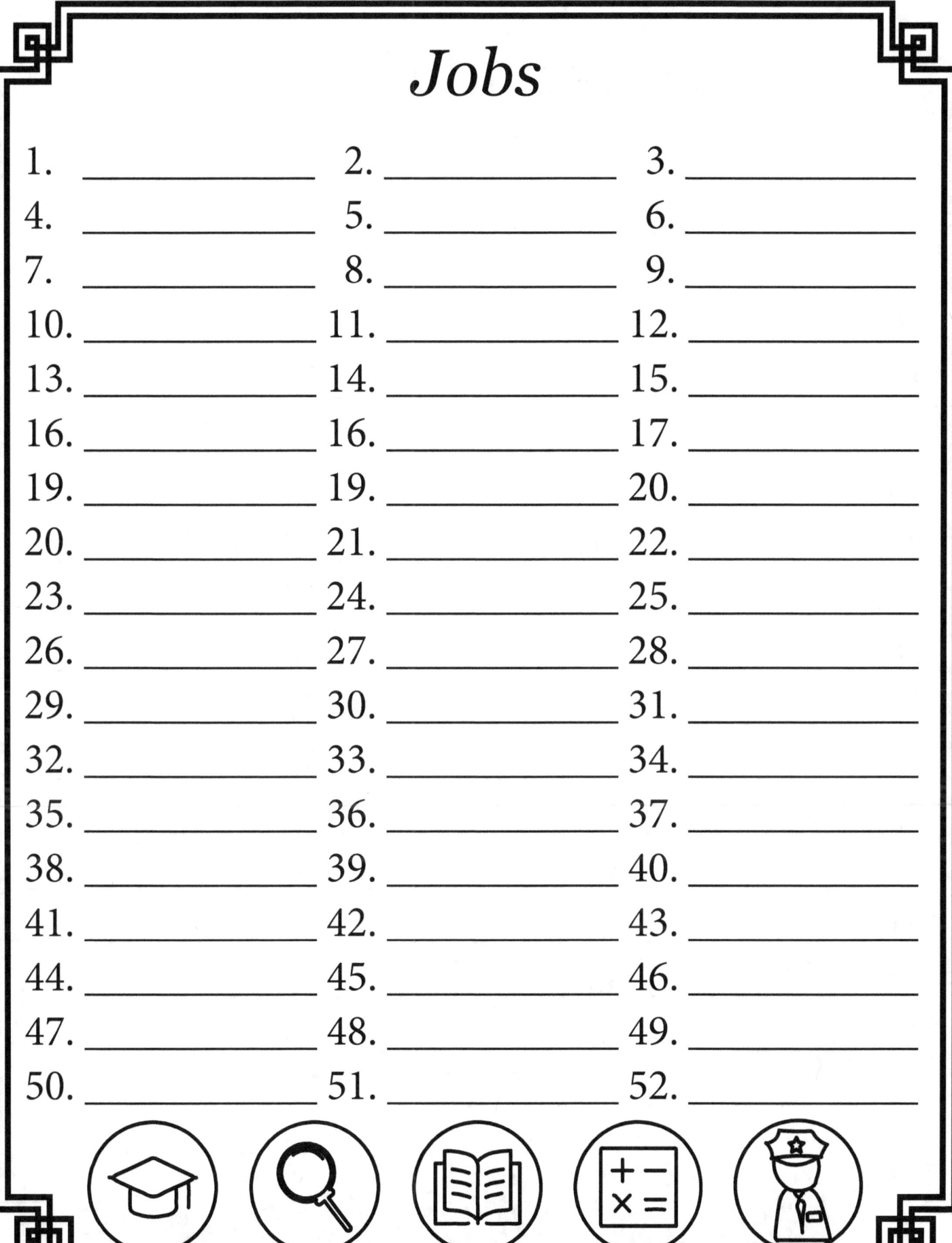

Fruits and Veggies

1. _____
2. _____
3. _____
4. _____
5. _____
6. _____
7. _____
8. _____
9. _____
10. _____
11. _____
12. _____
13. _____
14. _____
15. _____
16. _____
16. _____
17. _____
19. _____
19. _____
20. _____
20. _____
21. _____
22. _____
23. _____
24. _____
25. _____
26. _____
27. _____
28. _____
29. _____
30. _____
31. _____
32. _____
33. _____
34. _____
35. _____
36. _____
37. _____
38. _____
39. _____
40. _____
41. _____
42. _____
43. _____
44. _____
45. _____
46. _____
47. _____
48. _____
49. _____
50. _____
51. _____
52. _____

Animals

1. _____   2. _____   3. _____

4. _____   5. _____   6. _____

7. _____   8. _____   9. _____

10. _____   11. _____   12. _____

13. _____   14. _____   15. _____

16. _____   16. _____   17. _____

19. _____   19. _____   20. _____

20. _____   21. _____   22. _____

23. _____   24. _____   25. _____

26. _____   27. _____   28. _____

29. _____   30. _____   31. _____

32. _____   33. _____   34. _____

35. _____   36. _____   37. _____

38. _____   39. _____   40. _____

41. _____   42. _____   43. _____

44. _____   45. _____   46. _____

47. _____   48. _____   49. _____

50. _____   51. _____   52. _____

Cities

1. _____
2. _____
3. _____
4. _____
5. _____
6. _____
7. _____
8. _____
9. _____
10. _____
11. _____
12. _____
13. _____
14. _____
15. _____
16. _____
16. _____
17. _____
19. _____
19. _____
20. _____
20. _____
21. _____
22. _____
23. _____
24. _____
25. _____
26. _____
27. _____
28. _____
29. _____
30. _____
31. _____
32. _____
33. _____
34. _____
35. _____
36. _____
37. _____
38. _____
39. _____
40. _____
41. _____
42. _____
43. _____
44. _____
45. _____
46. _____
47. _____
48. _____
49. _____
50. _____
51. _____
52. _____

Weather

1. _____
2. _____
3. _____
4. _____
5. _____
6. _____
7. _____
8. _____
9. _____
10. _____
11. _____
12. _____
13. _____
14. _____
15. _____
16. _____
16. _____
17. _____
19. _____
19. _____
20. _____
20. _____
21. _____
22. _____
23. _____
24. _____
25. _____
26. _____
27. _____
28. _____
29. _____
30. _____
31. _____
32. _____
33. _____
34. _____
35. _____
36. _____
37. _____
38. _____
39. _____
40. _____
41. _____
42. _____
43. _____
44. _____
45. _____
46. _____
47. _____
48. _____
49. _____
50. _____
51. _____
52. _____

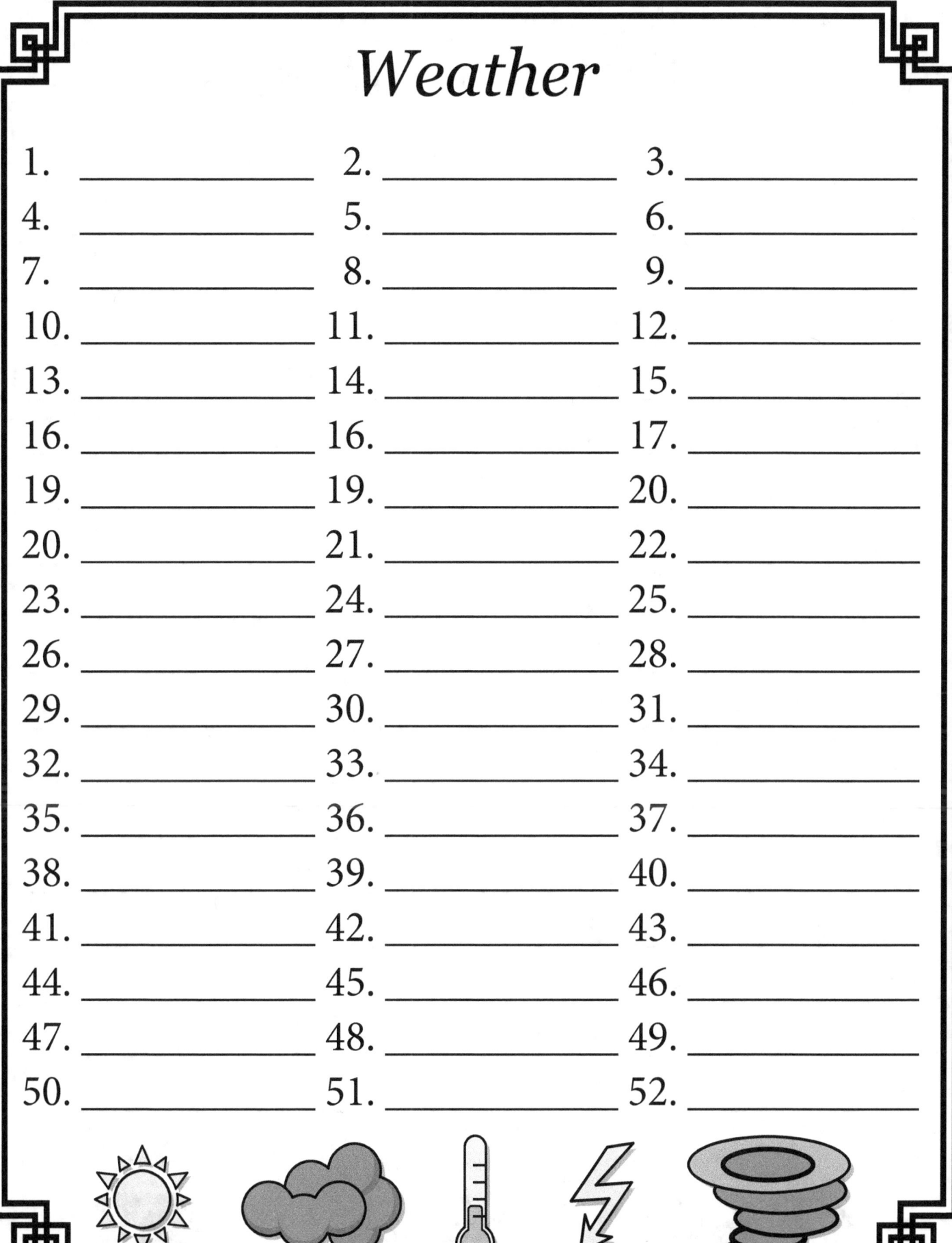

Transportation

1. _____   2. _____   3. _____
4. _____   5. _____   6. _____
7. _____   8. _____   9. _____
10. _____   11. _____   12. _____
13. _____   14. _____   15. _____
16. _____   16. _____   17. _____
19. _____   19. _____   20. _____
20. _____   21. _____   22. _____
23. _____   24. _____   25. _____
26. _____   27. _____   28. _____
29. _____   30. _____   31. _____
32. _____   33. _____   34. _____
35. _____   36. _____   37. _____
38. _____   39. _____   40. _____
41. _____   42. _____   43. _____
44. _____   45. _____   46. _____
47. _____   48. _____   49. _____
50. _____   51. _____   52. _____

Hobbies

1. _____
2. _____
3. _____
4. _____
5. _____
6. _____
7. _____
8. _____
9. _____
10. _____
11. _____
12. _____
13. _____
14. _____
15. _____
16. _____
16. _____
17. _____
19. _____
19. _____
20. _____
20. _____
21. _____
22. _____
23. _____
24. _____
25. _____
26. _____
27. _____
28. _____
29. _____
30. _____
31. _____
32. _____
33. _____
34. _____
35. _____
36. _____
37. _____
38. _____
39. _____
40. _____
41. _____
42. _____
43. _____
44. _____
45. _____
46. _____
47. _____
48. _____
49. _____
50. _____
51. _____
52. _____

Examples

Cooking

1. pot
2. pan
3. ingredients
4. salt
5. spices
6. oven
7. knives
8. dicing
9. chopping

Sports

1. baseball
2. basketball
3. golf
4. tennis
5. hockey
6. gymnastics
7. track
8. field
9. goal

Summer

1. hot
2. sun
3. beach
4. vacation
5. sunglasses
6. tan
7. bathing suit
8. August
9. picnic

Jobs

1. police officer
2. fire fighter
3. secretary
4. postal worker
5. teacher
6. boss
7. HR
8. cashier
9. janitor

Examples

Fruits and Veggies

1. strawberries
2. celery
3. apples
4. lettuce
5. kiwi
6. oranges
7. carrots
8. leeks
9. watermelon

Animals

1. elephants
2. giraffes
3. dogs
4. cows
5. chickens
6. rhinos
7. hippos
8. zebra
9. deer

Cities

1. New York
2. Chicago
3. New Delhi
4. Hong Kong
5. London
6. Paris
7. Cairo
8. Buenos Aires
9. Sydney

Weather

1. storm
2. sunny
3. rain
4. snow
5. wind
6. sleet
7. cloud
8. tornado
9. hurricane

Examples

Transportation

1. train
2. truck
3. car
4. plane
5. helicopter
6. van
7. Jeep
8. bicycle
9. scooter

Hobbies

1. photo
2. fishing
3. golf
4. sailing
5. painting
6. coin collecting
7. hiking
8. crafts
9. knitting

Find the Match

Draw a line connecting the matching objects, then circle the leftover object that doesn't match.

As an example, the first match is completed for you.

Find the Match: Fall

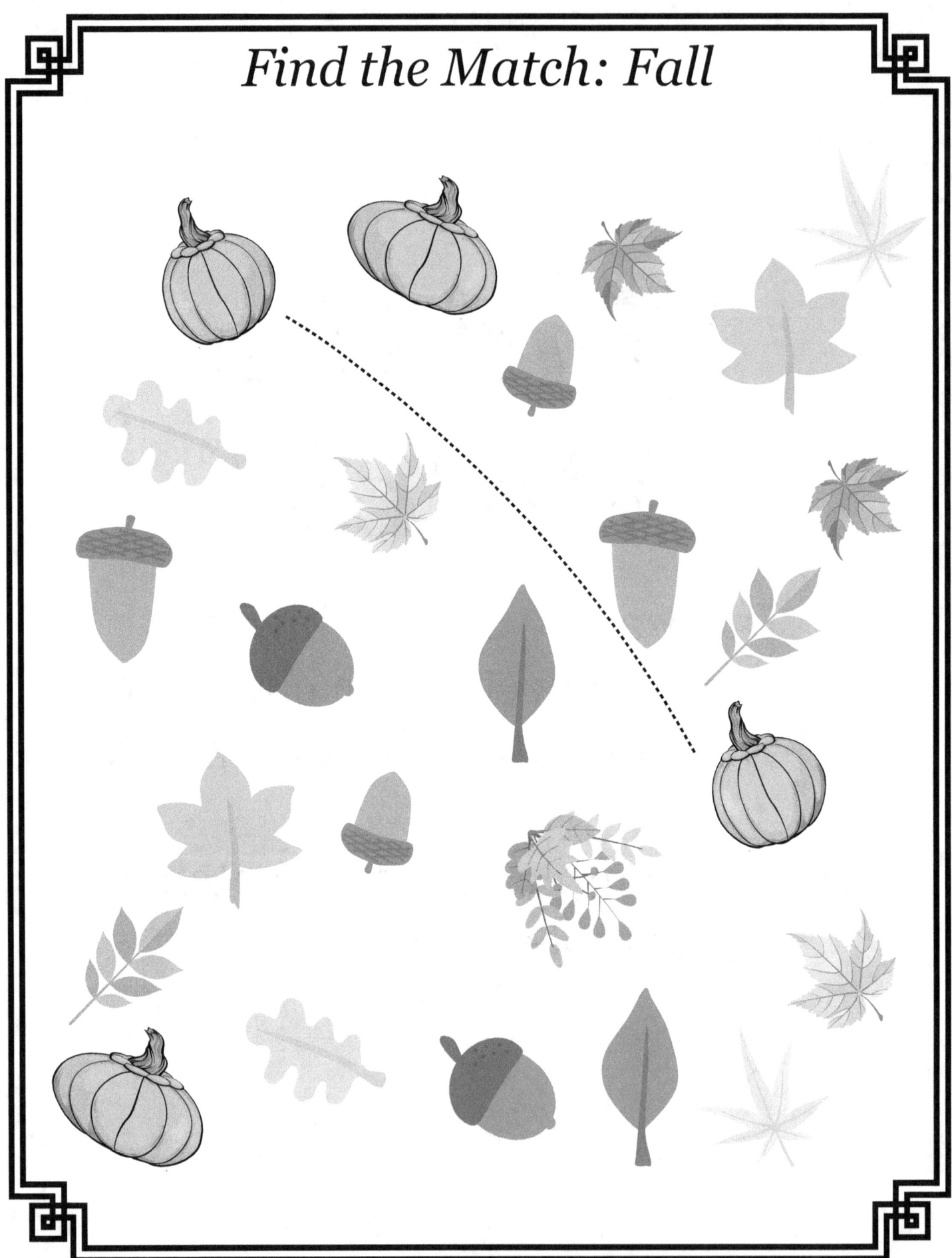

Find the Match: Dogs

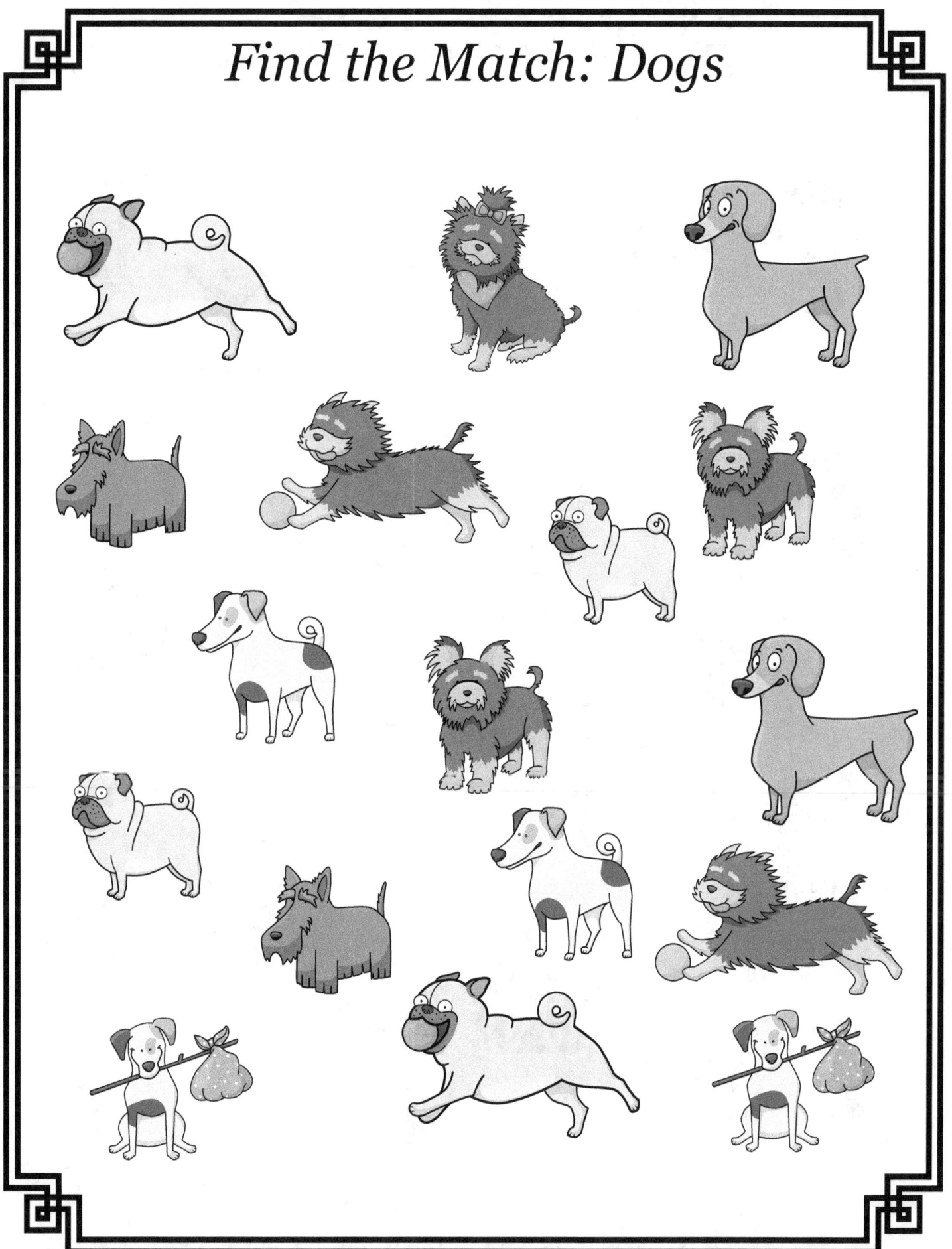

Find the Match: Circus

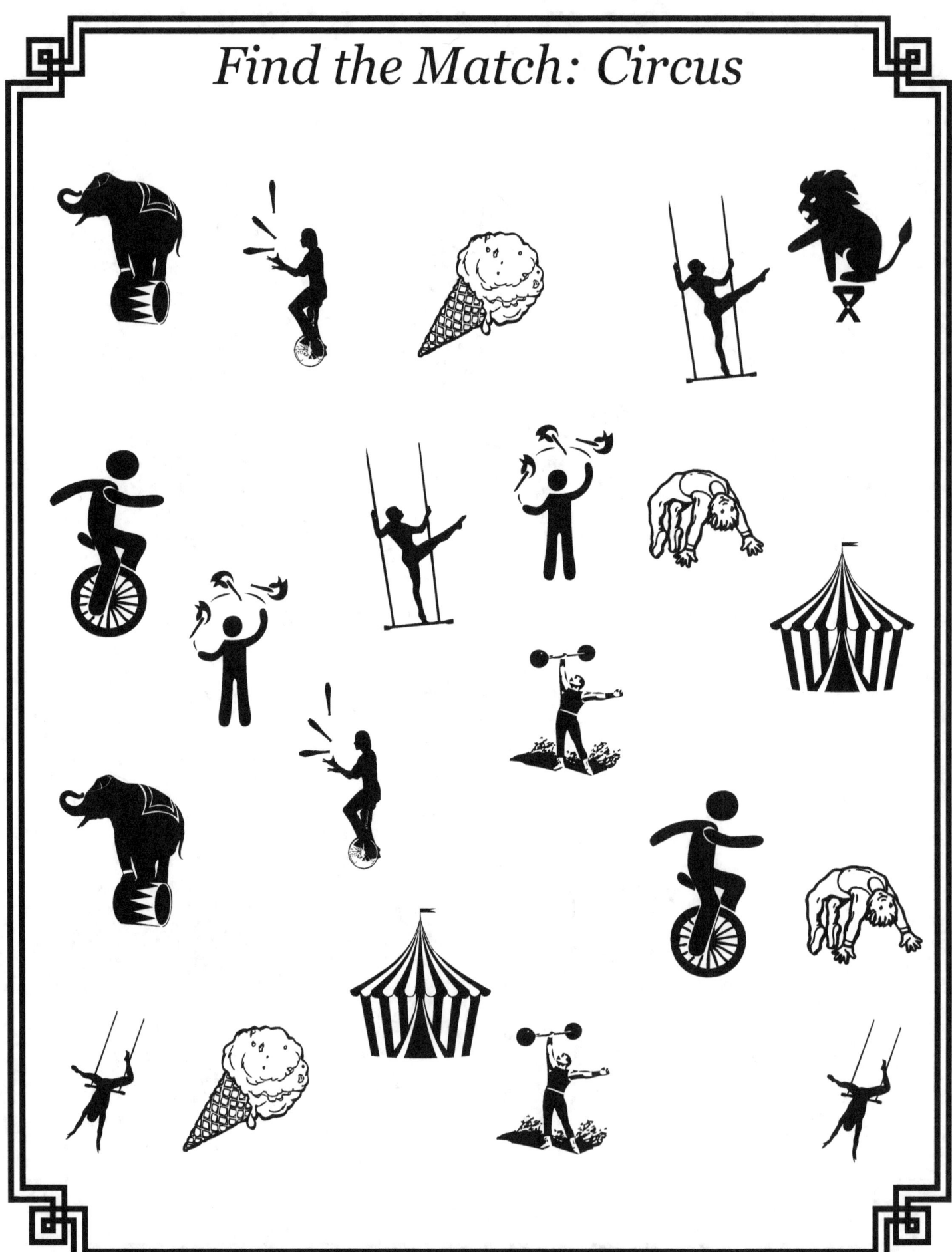

Find the Match: Birds

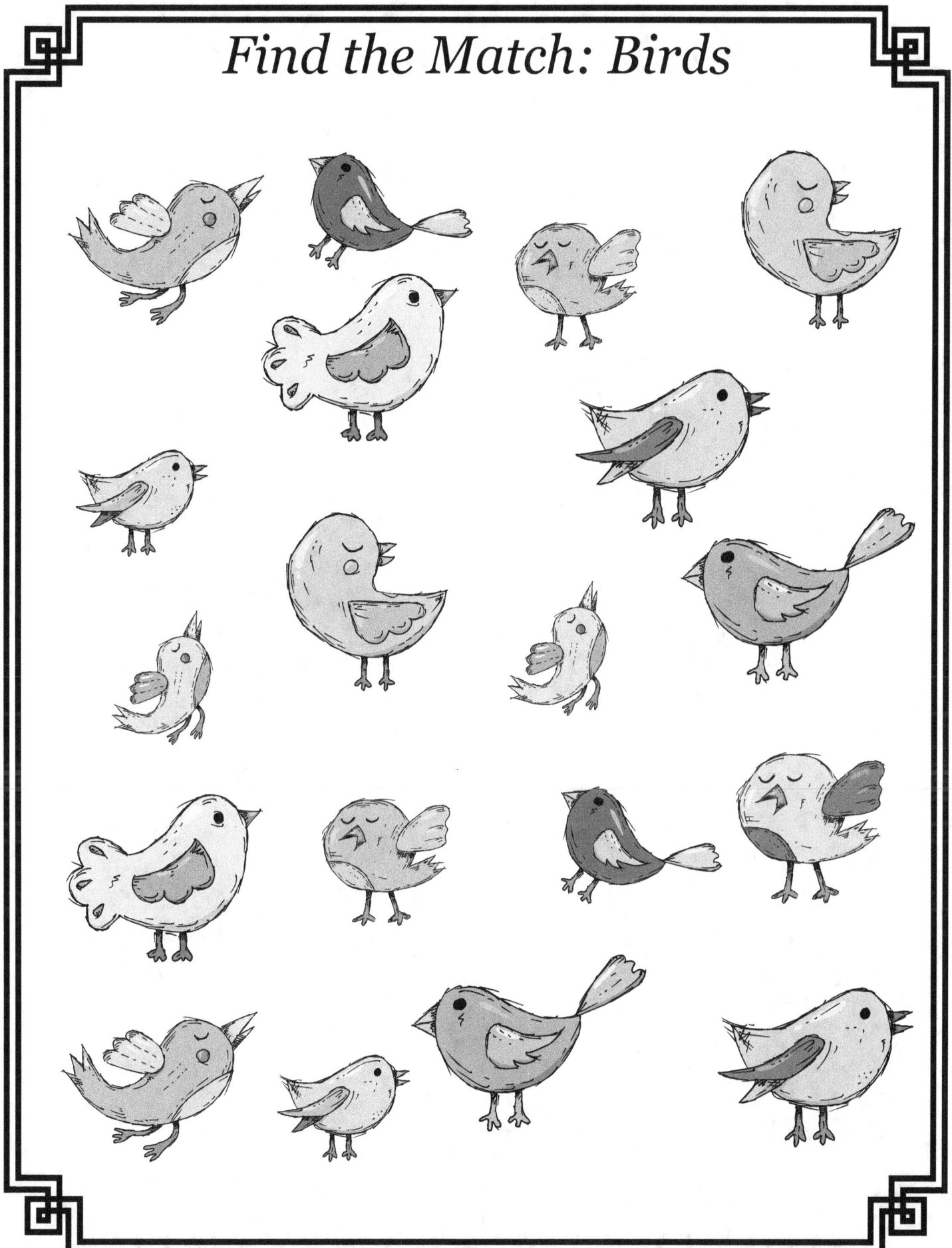

Find the Match: Donuts

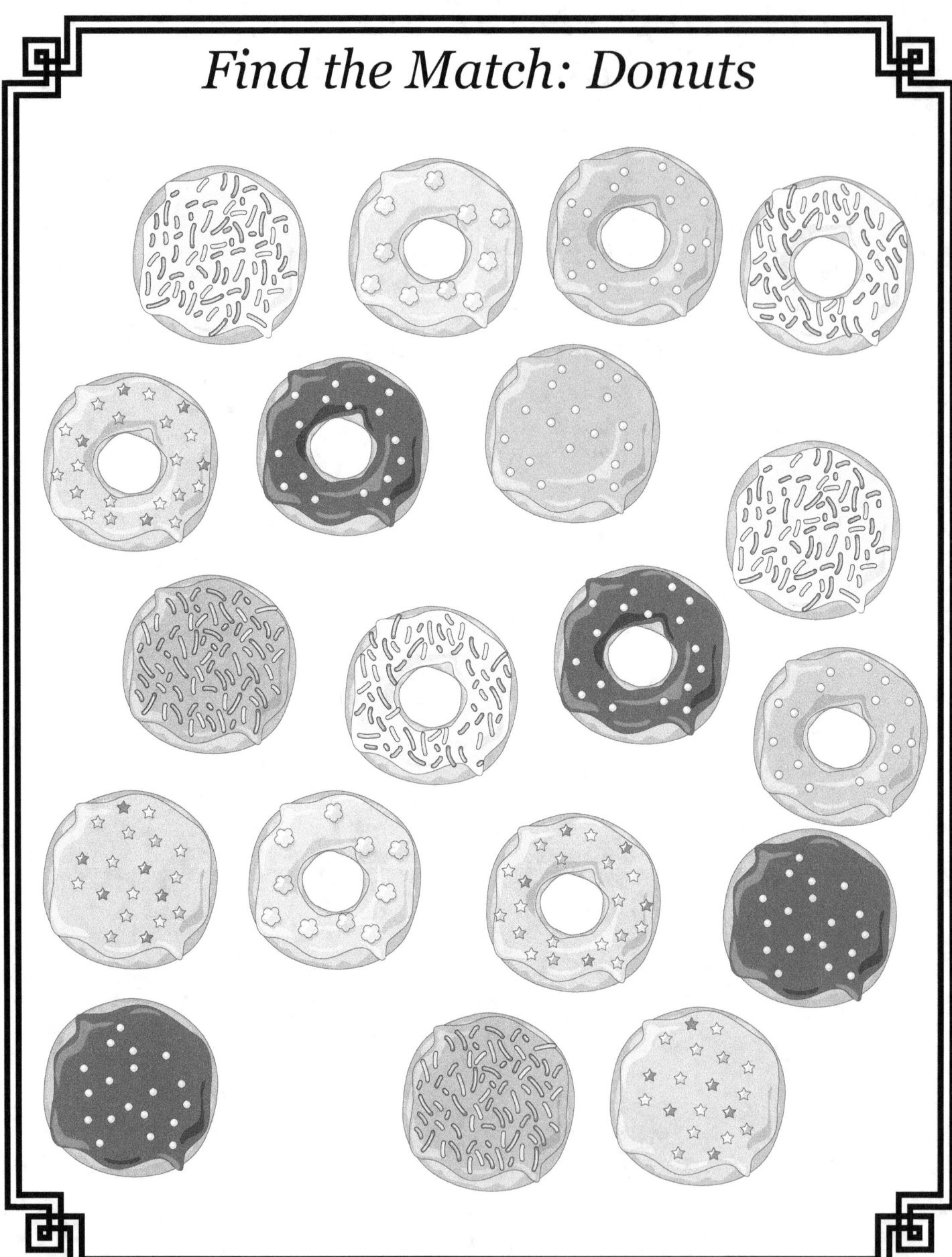

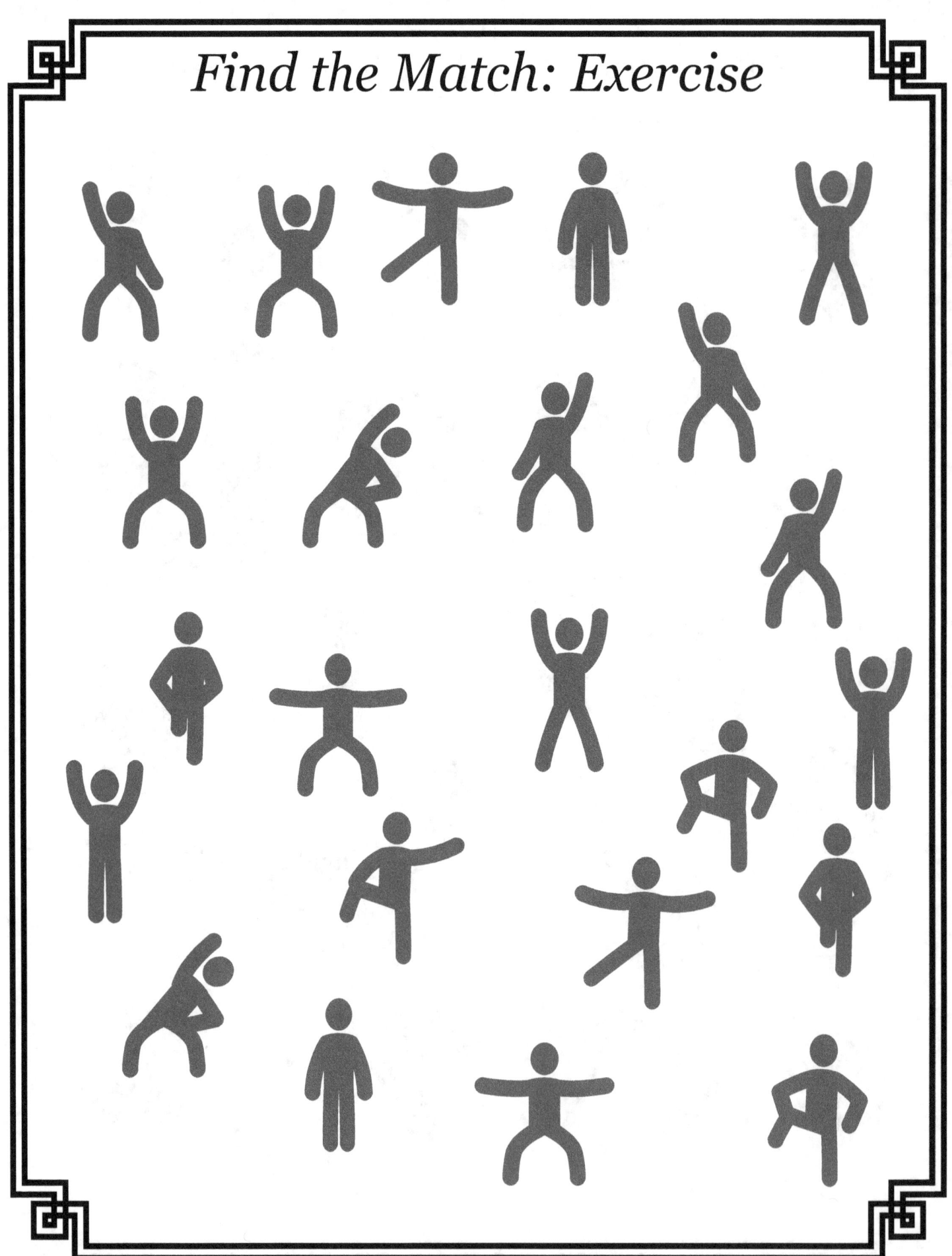

Find the Match: Zoo

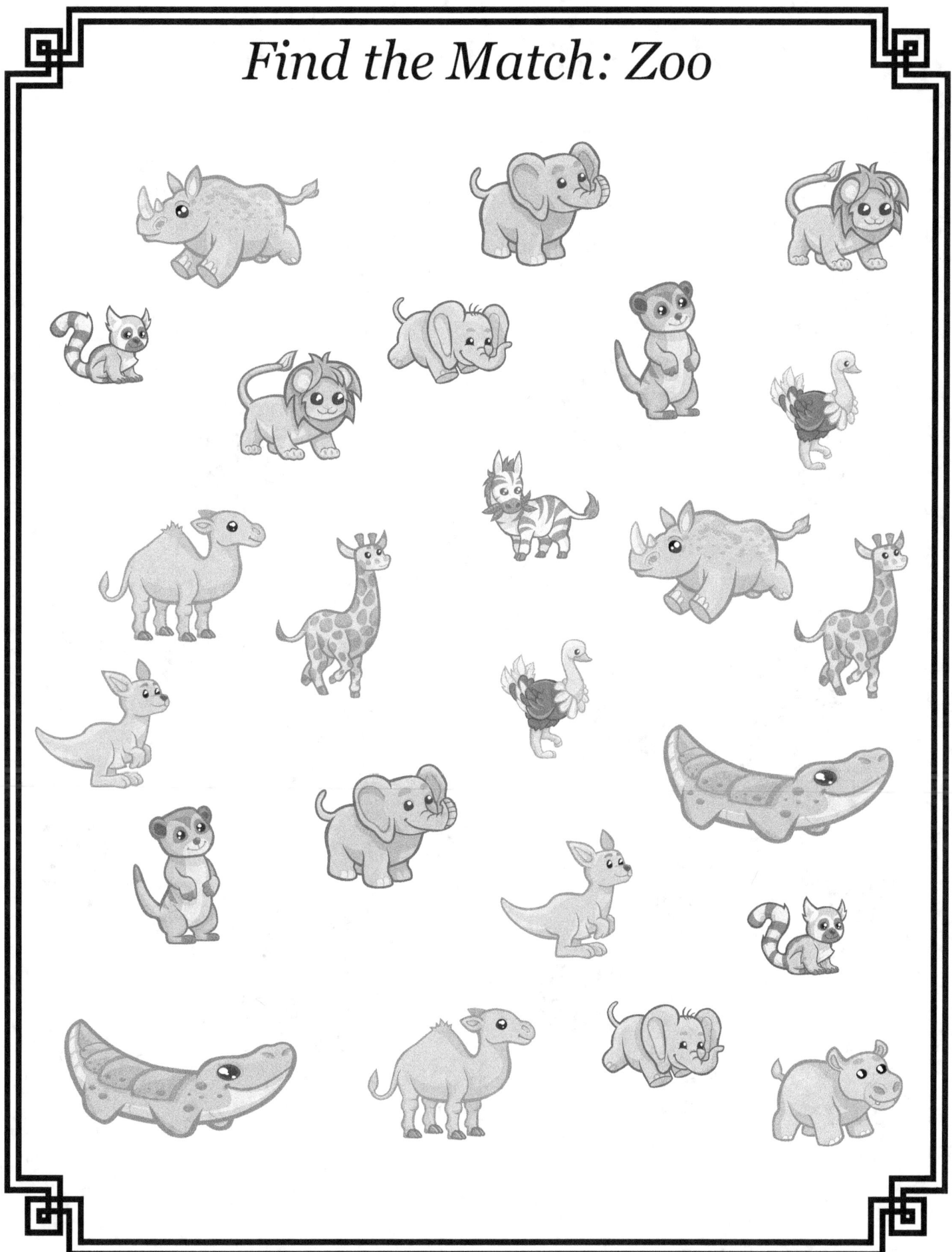

Find the Match: Snowflakes

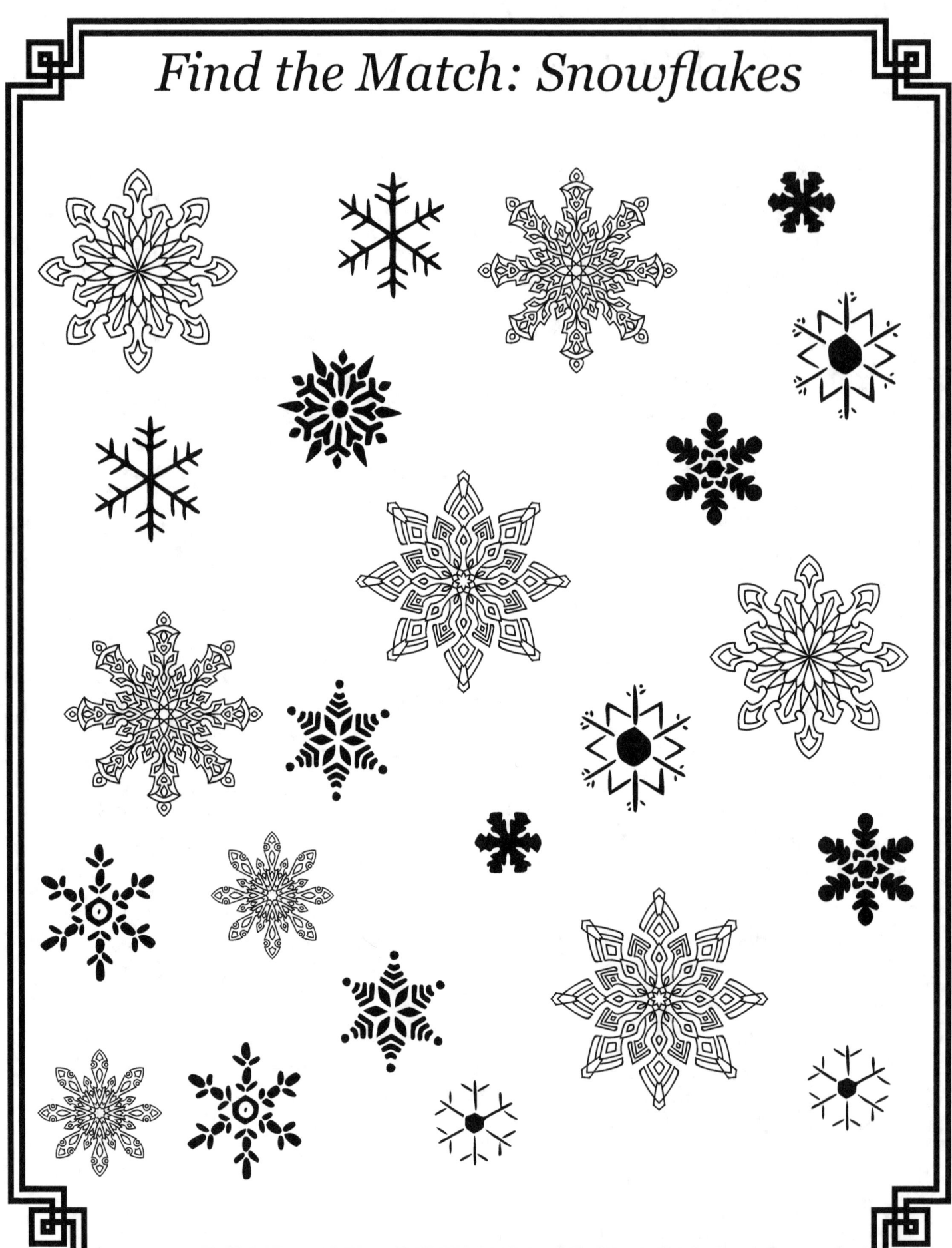

Find the Match: Music

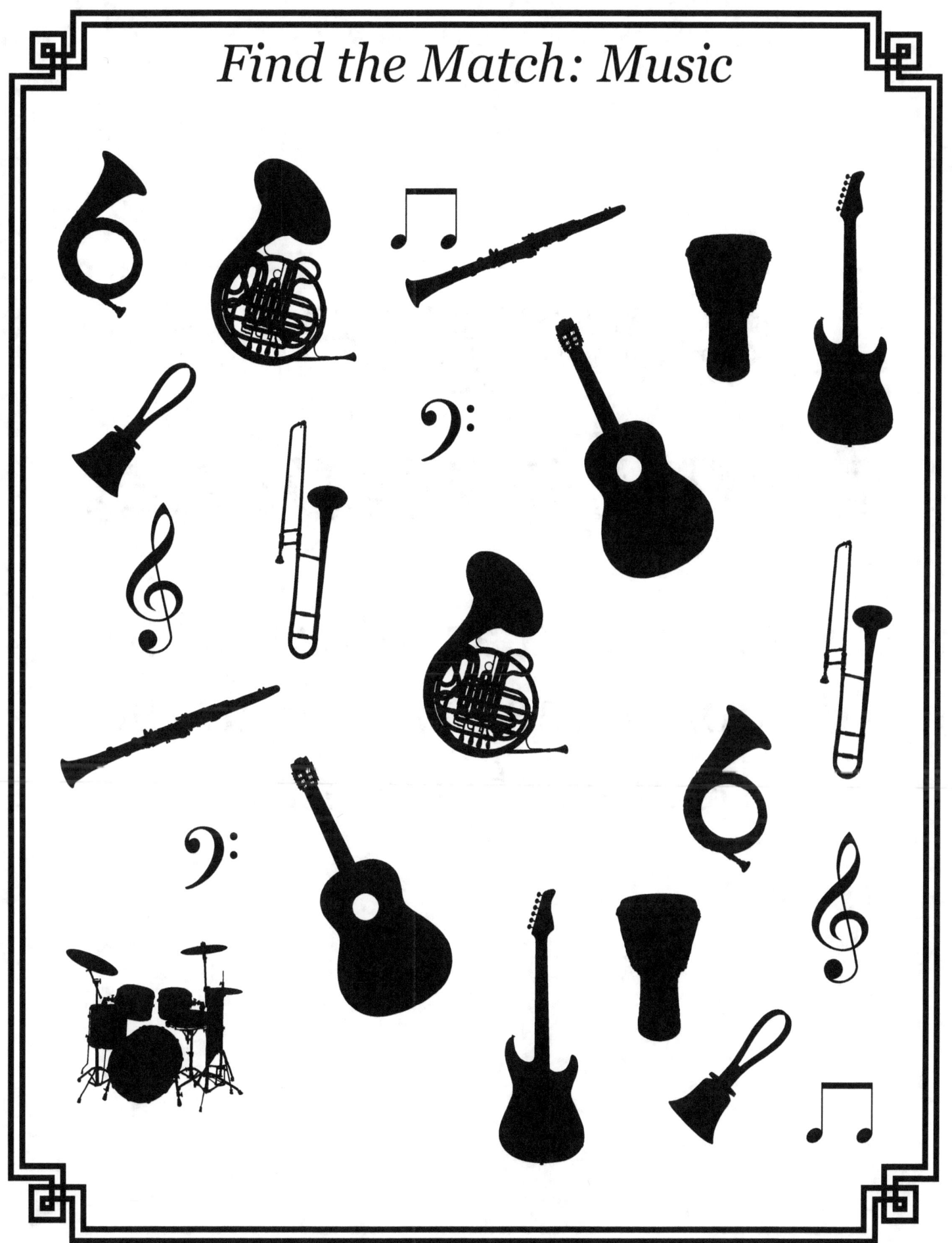

Complete the Drawing

Use the grid as reference to complete the drawing at the bottom of each page.

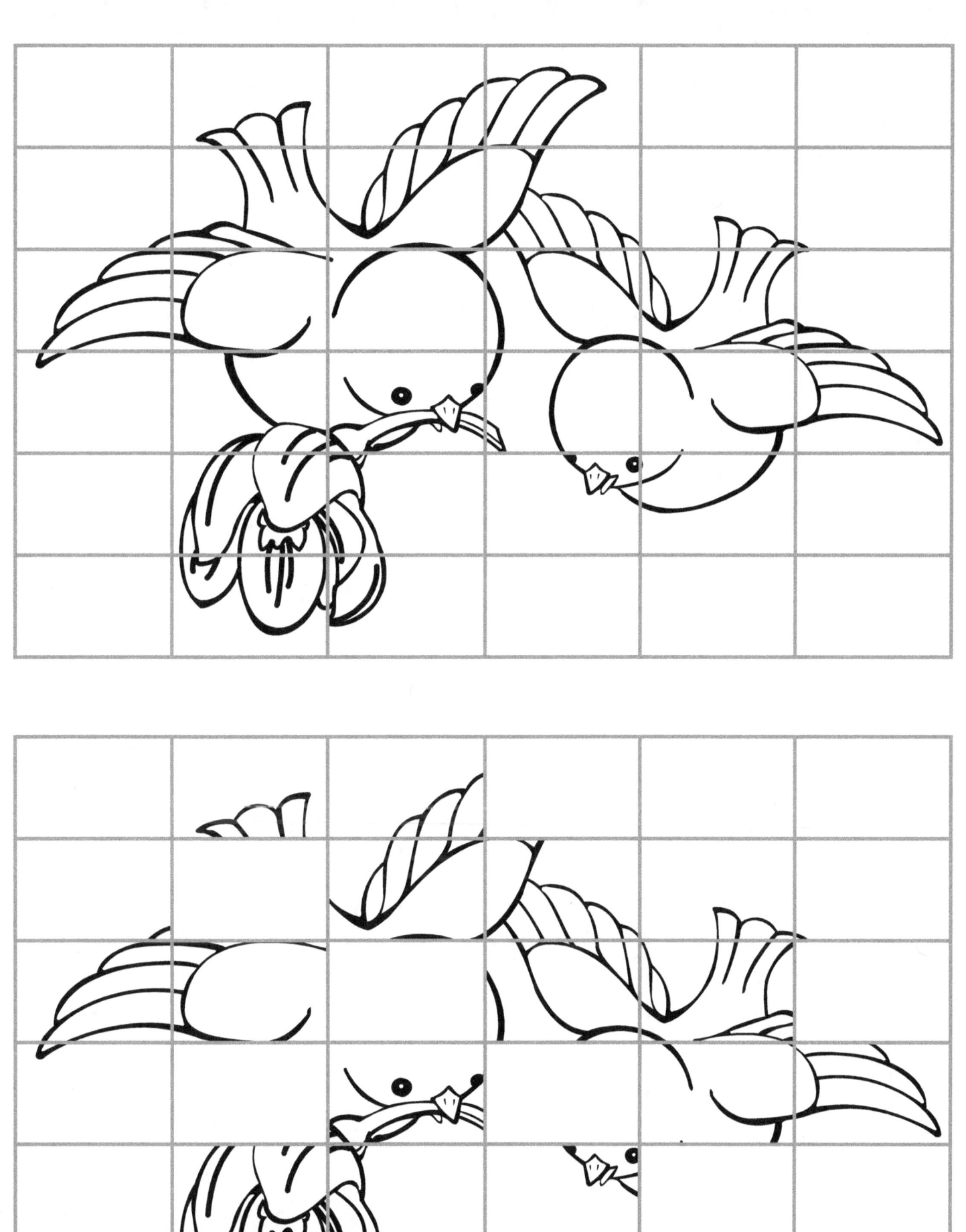

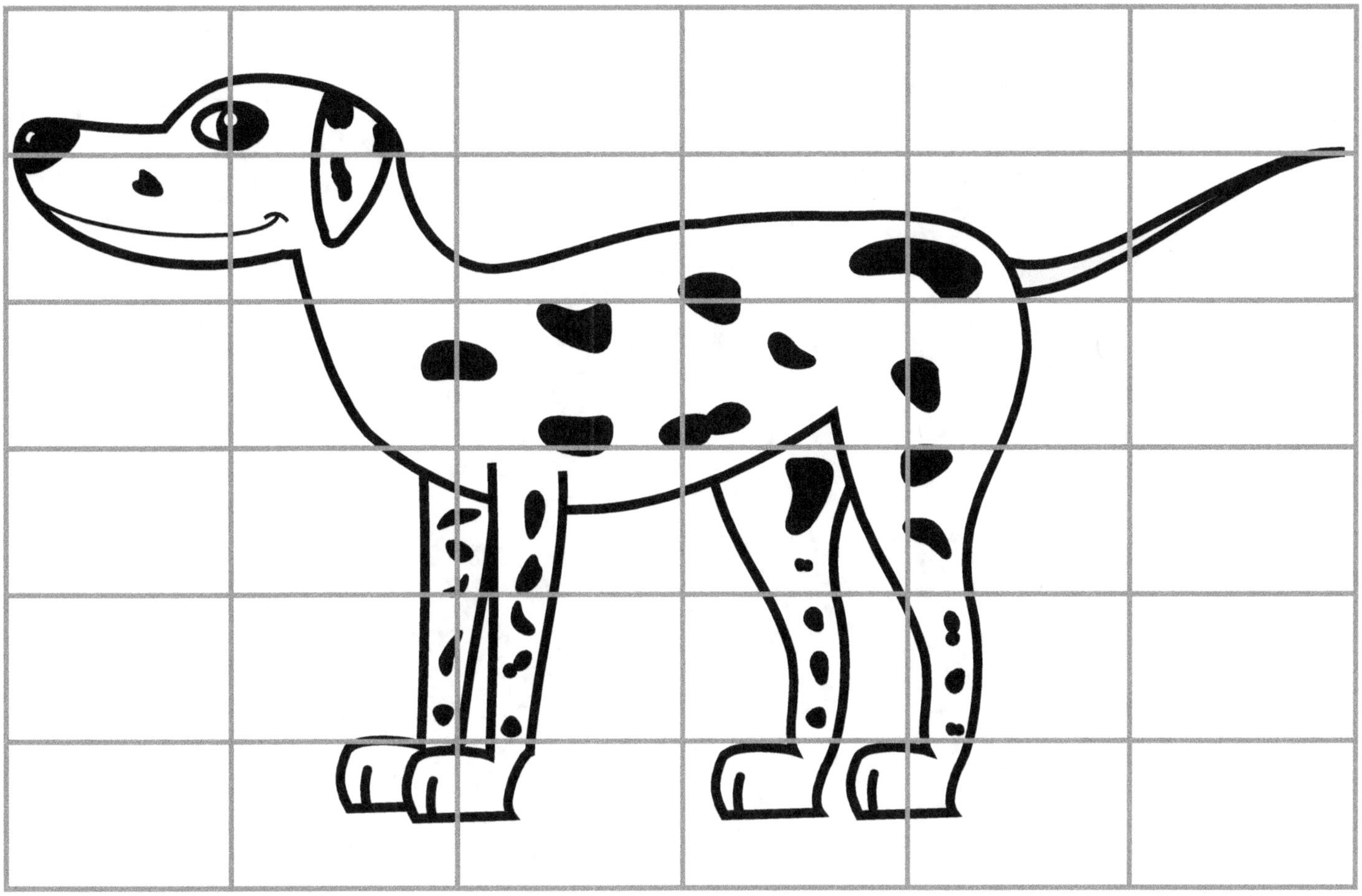

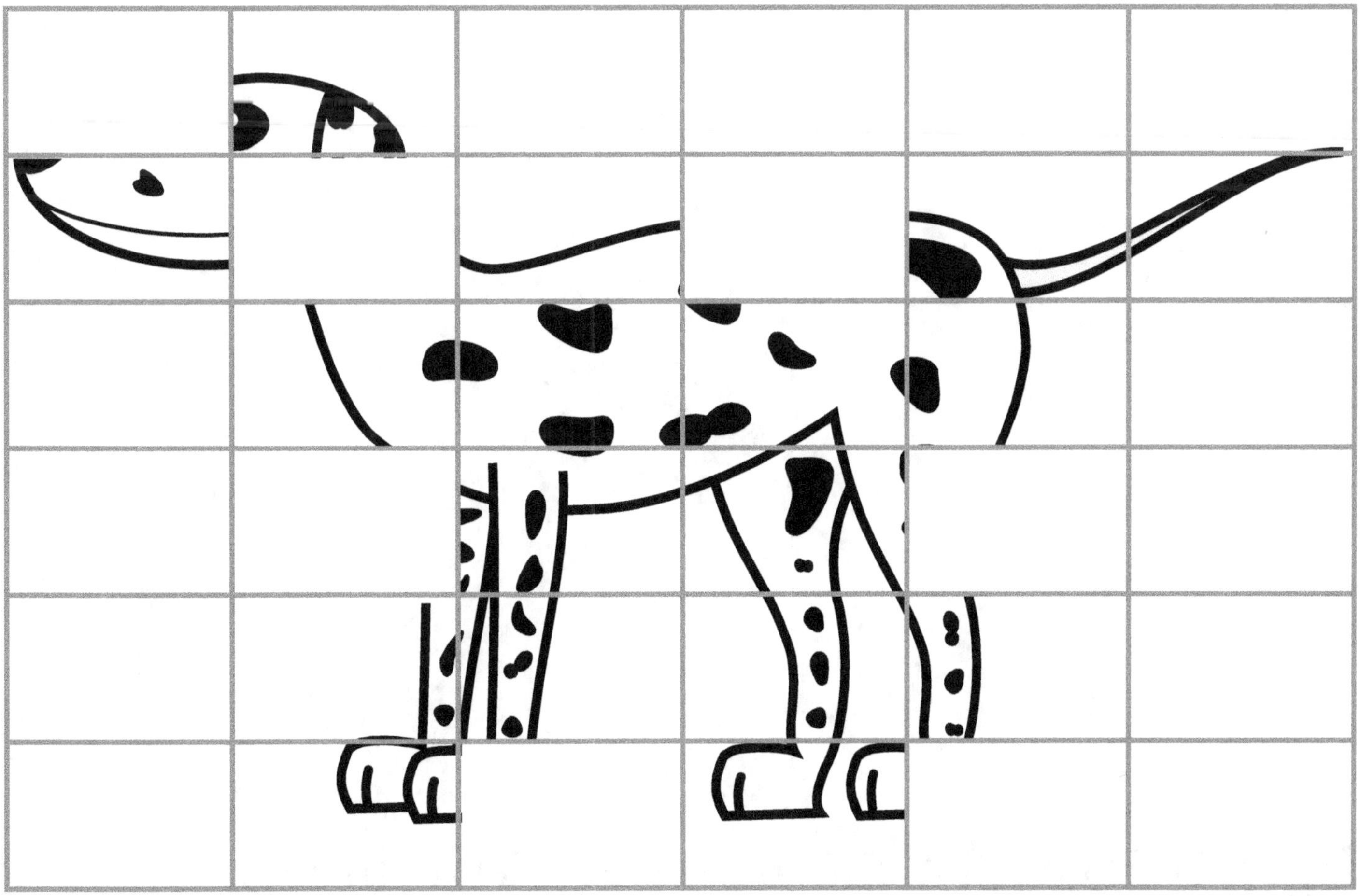

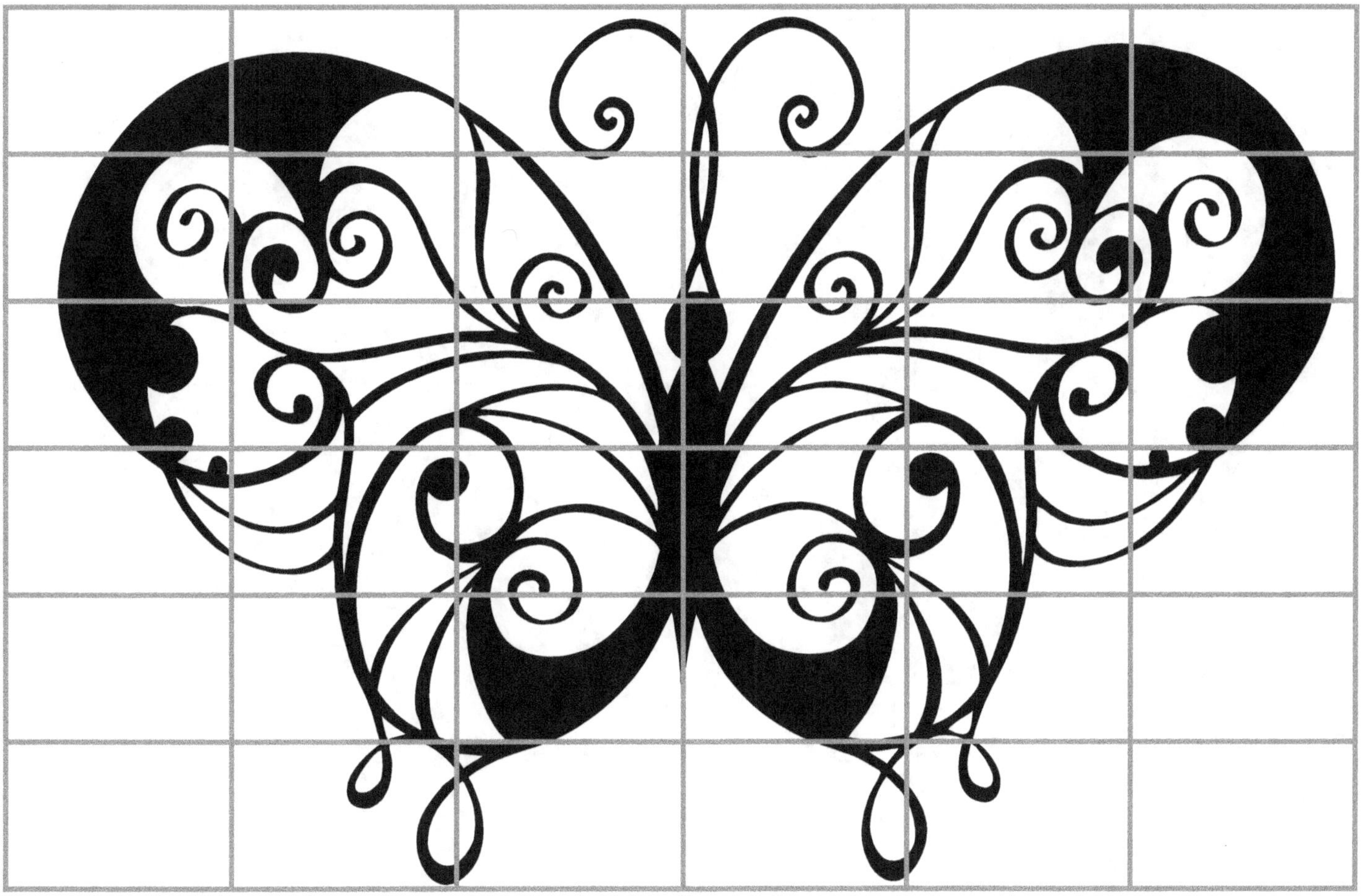

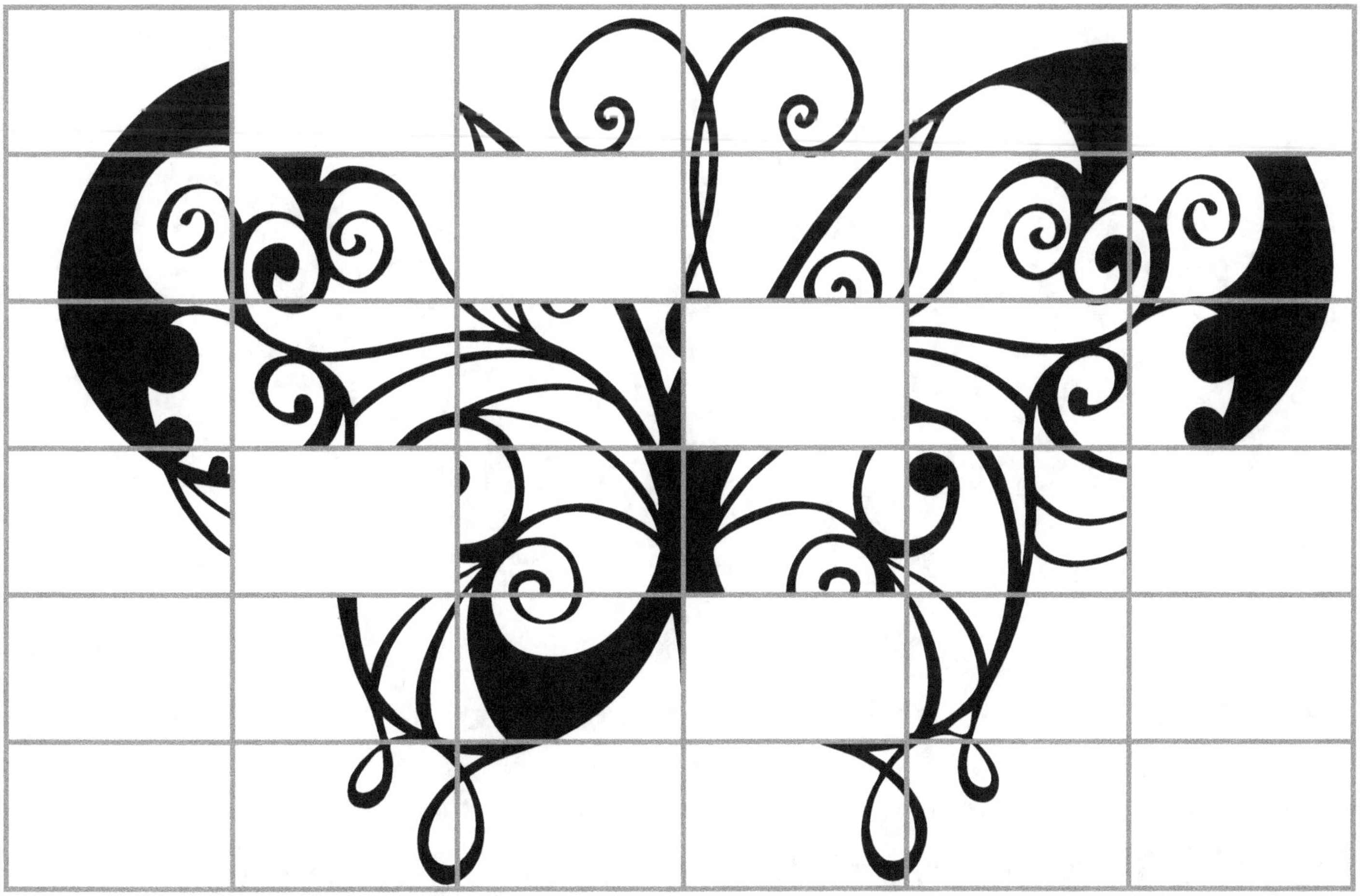

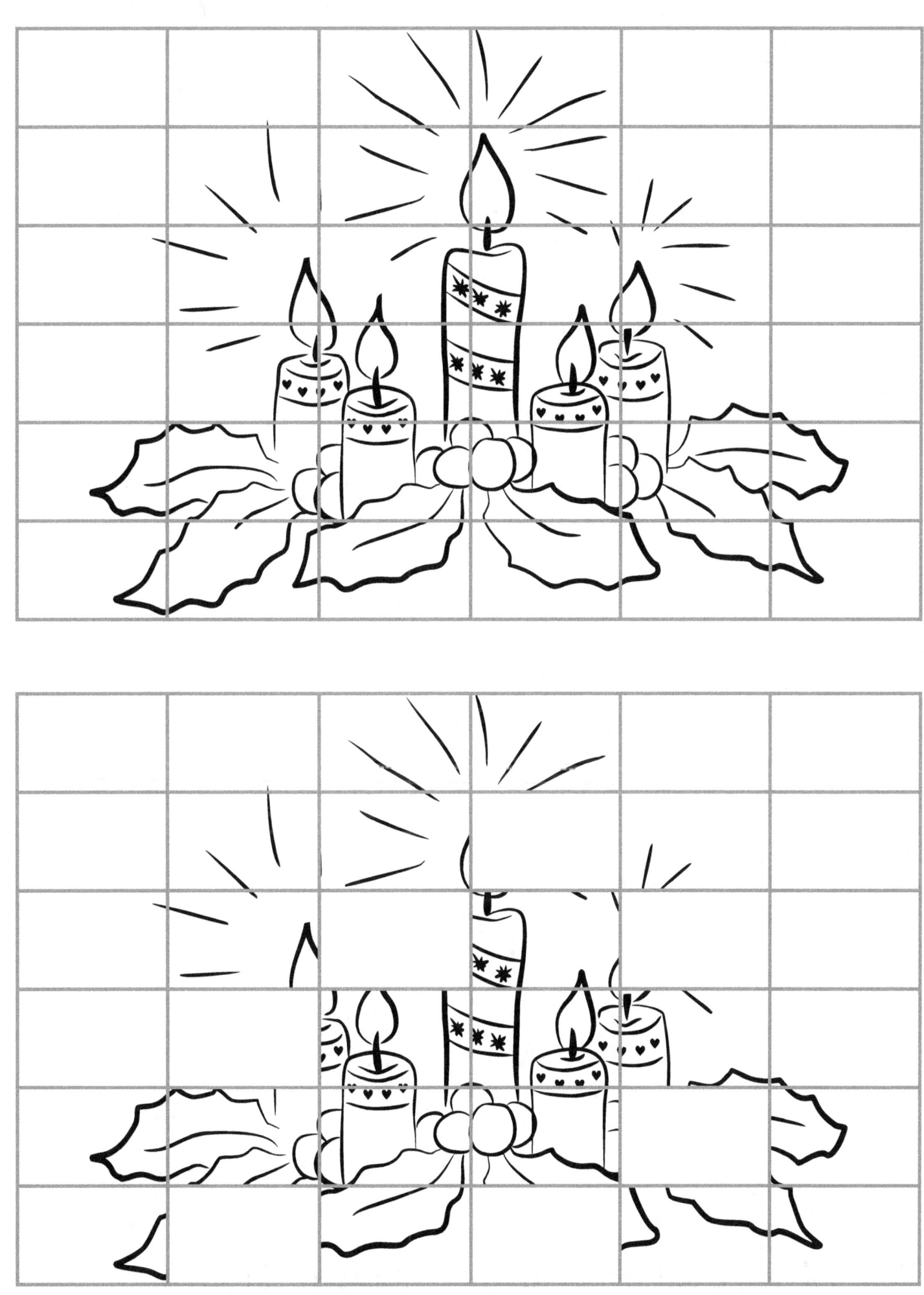

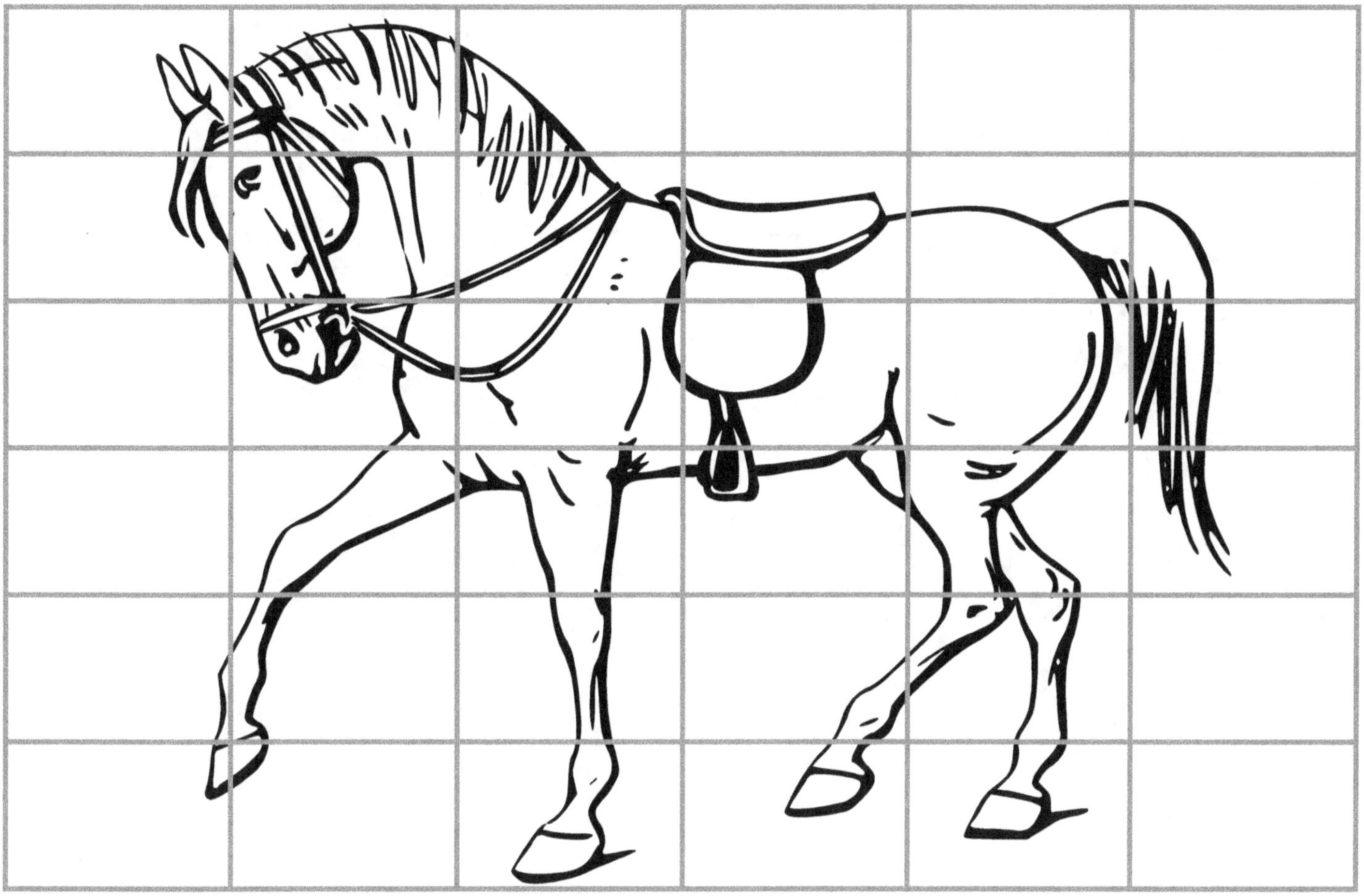

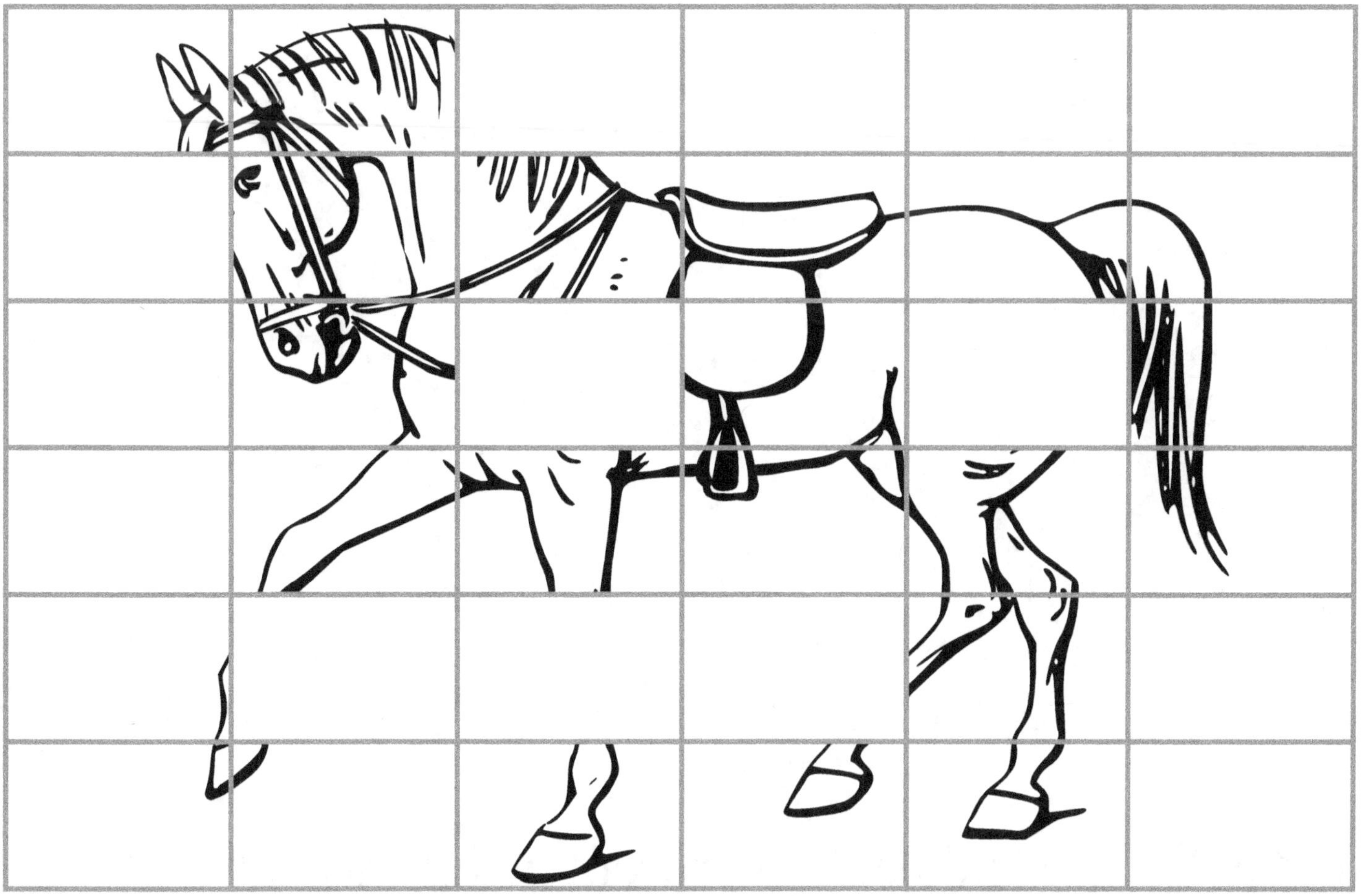

Pg. 96 Page left blank to prevent bleed-through.

How Many

How many of each image can you find? Write the number in the boxes at the bottom of the page.

How Many Cupcakes?

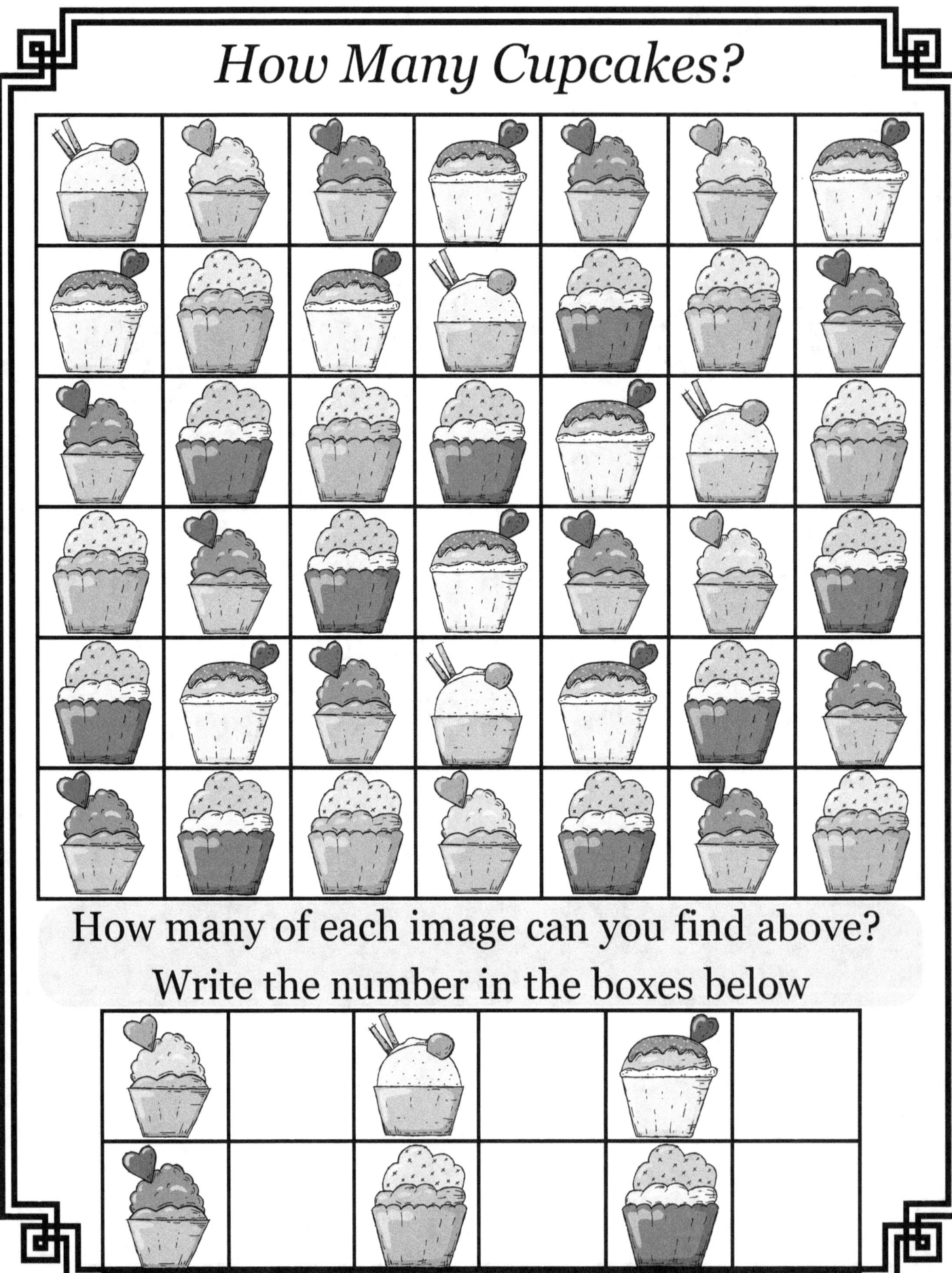

How many of each image can you find above?

Write the number in the boxes below

How Many Owls?

How many of each image can you find above?

Write the number in the boxes below

How Many Leaves?

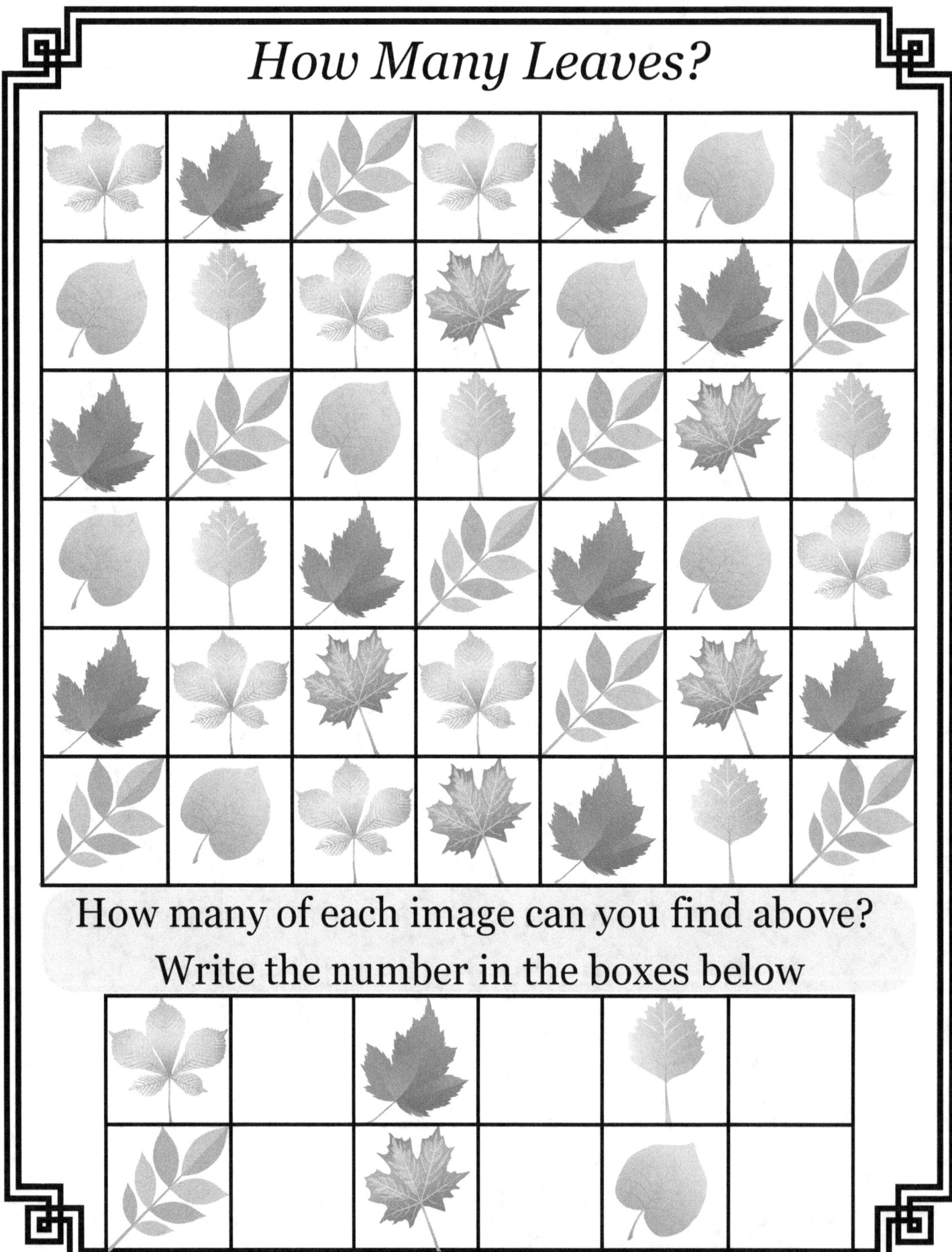

How many of each image can you find above?
Write the number in the boxes below

How Many Faces?

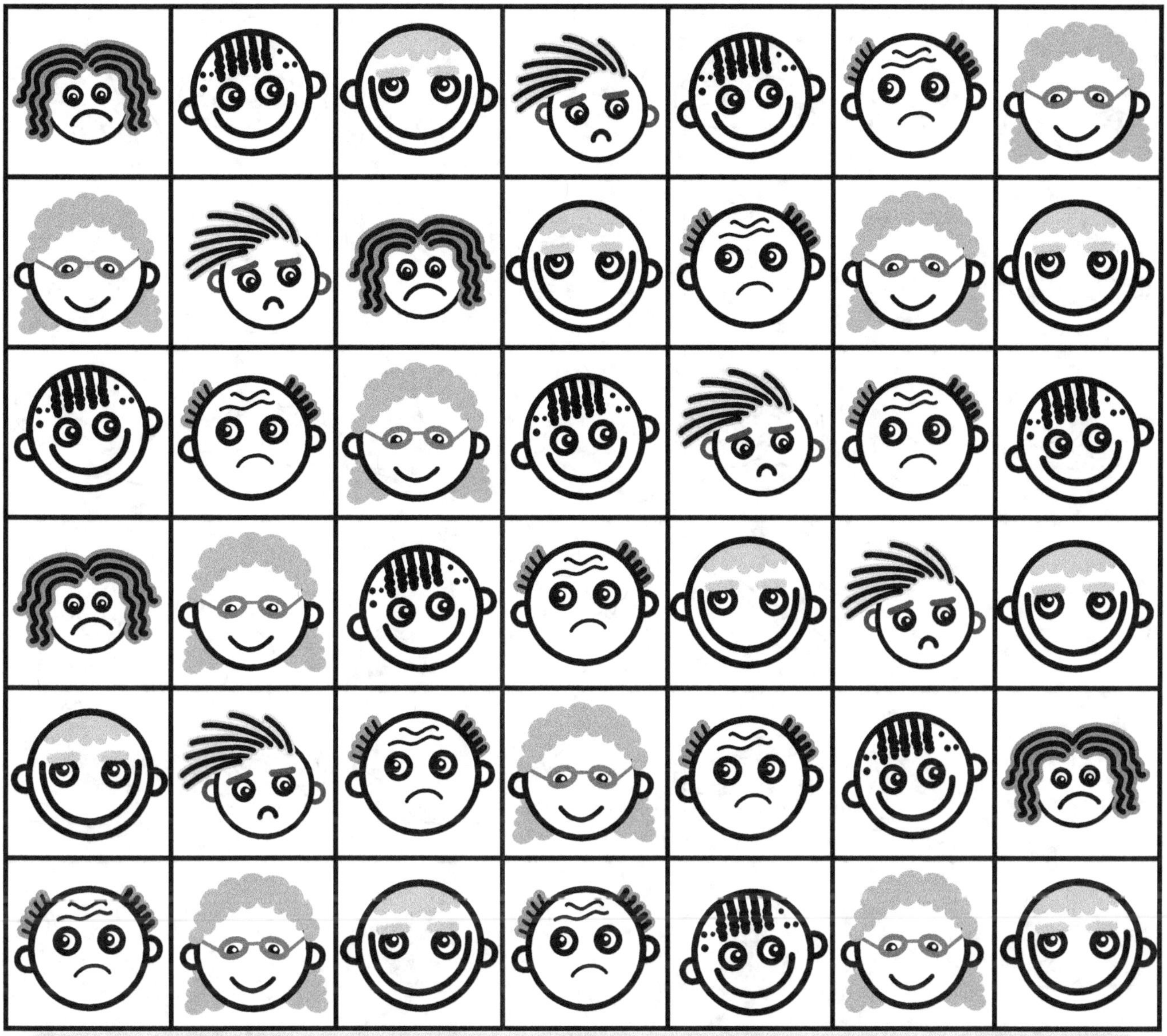

How many of each image can you find above?

Write the number in the boxes below

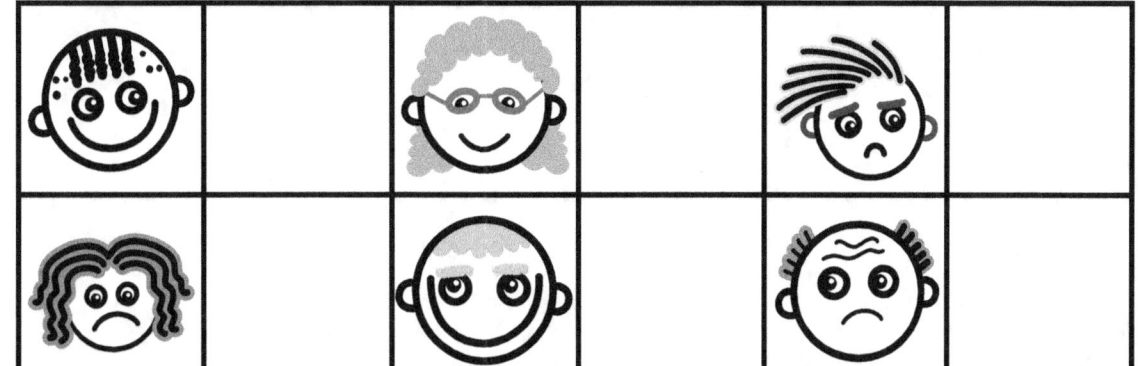

How Many Shoes?

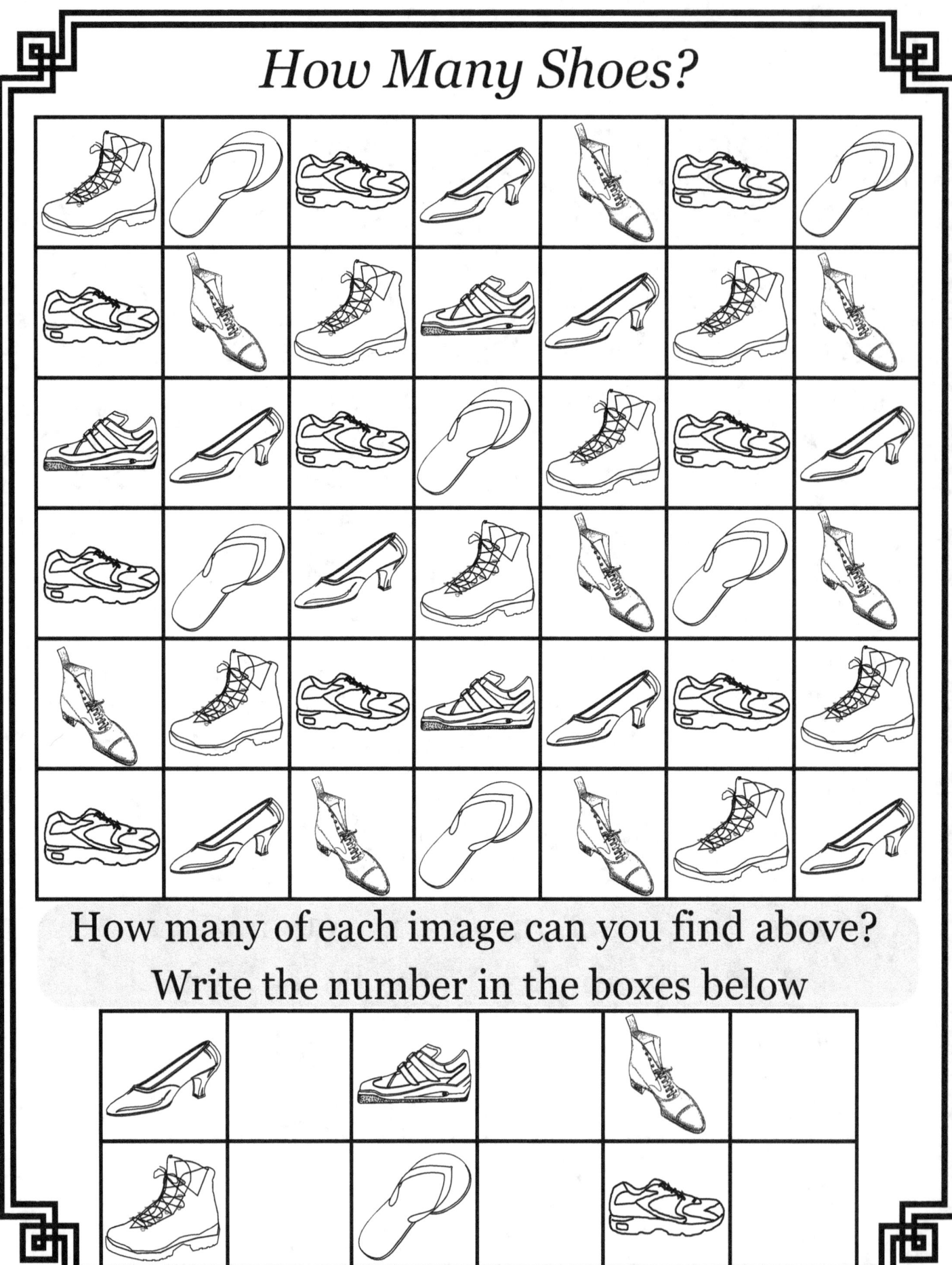

How many of each image can you find above?

Write the number in the boxes below

How Many Monkeys?

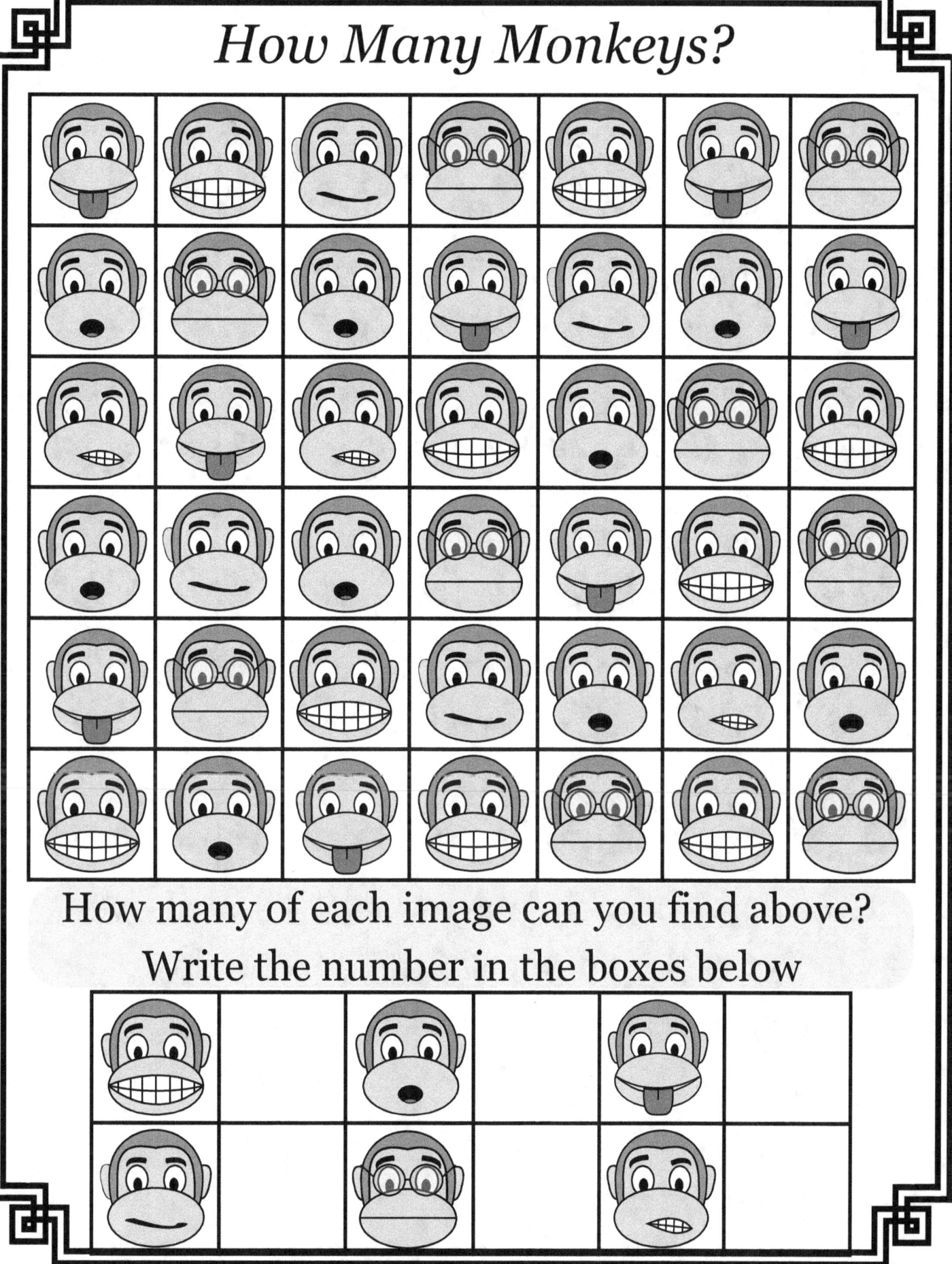

How many of each image can you find above?

Write the number in the boxes below

How Many Flowers?

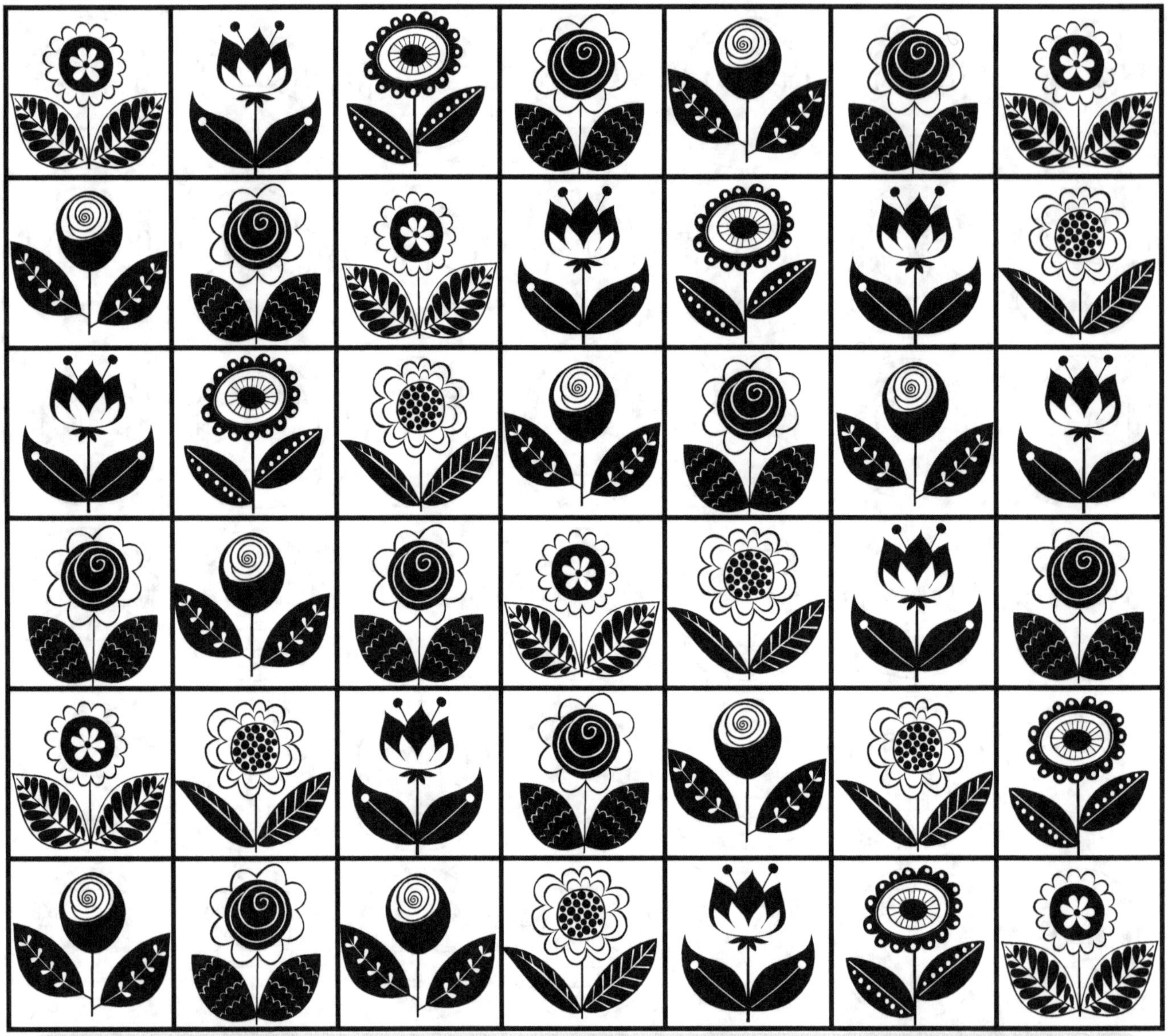

How many of each image can you find above?

Write the number in the boxes below

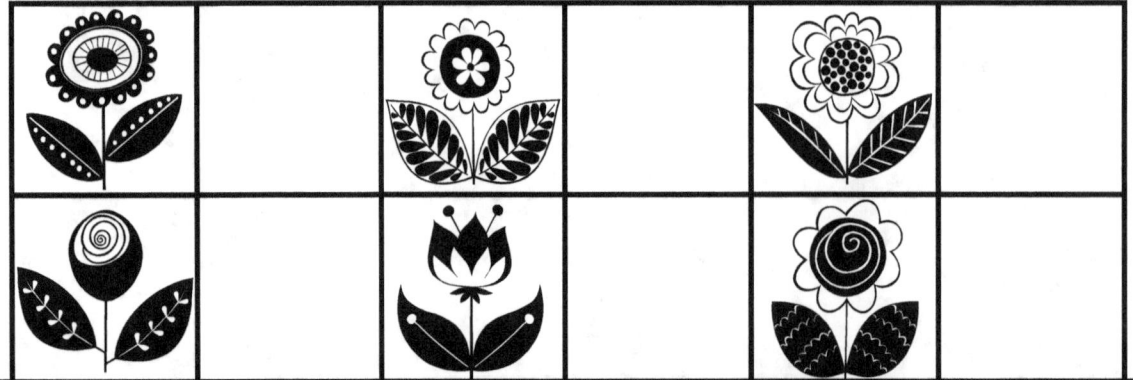

How Many Buttons?

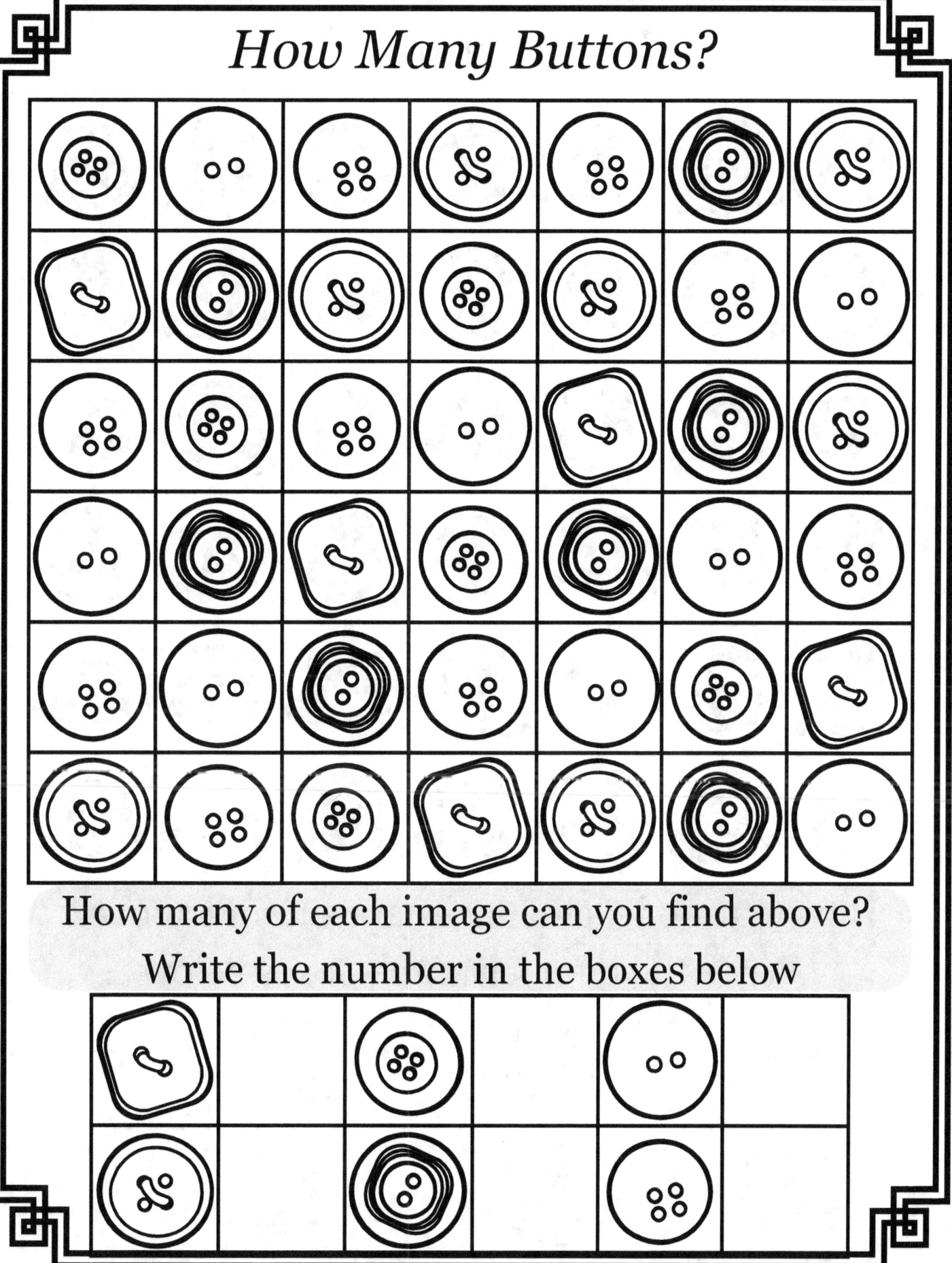

How many of each image can you find above?
Write the number in the boxes below

How Many Hats?

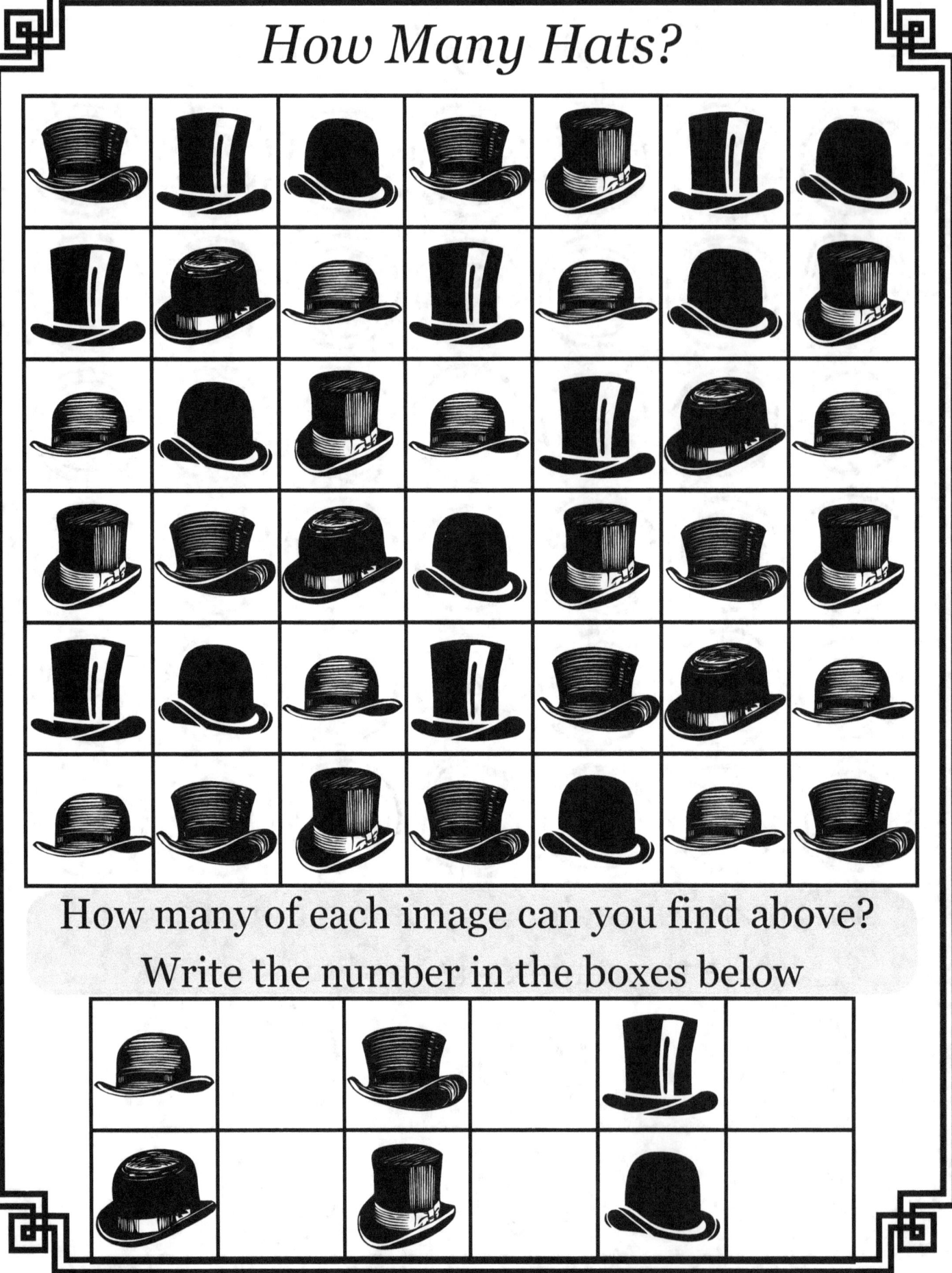

How many of each image can you find above?

Write the number in the boxes below

How Many Sunglasses?

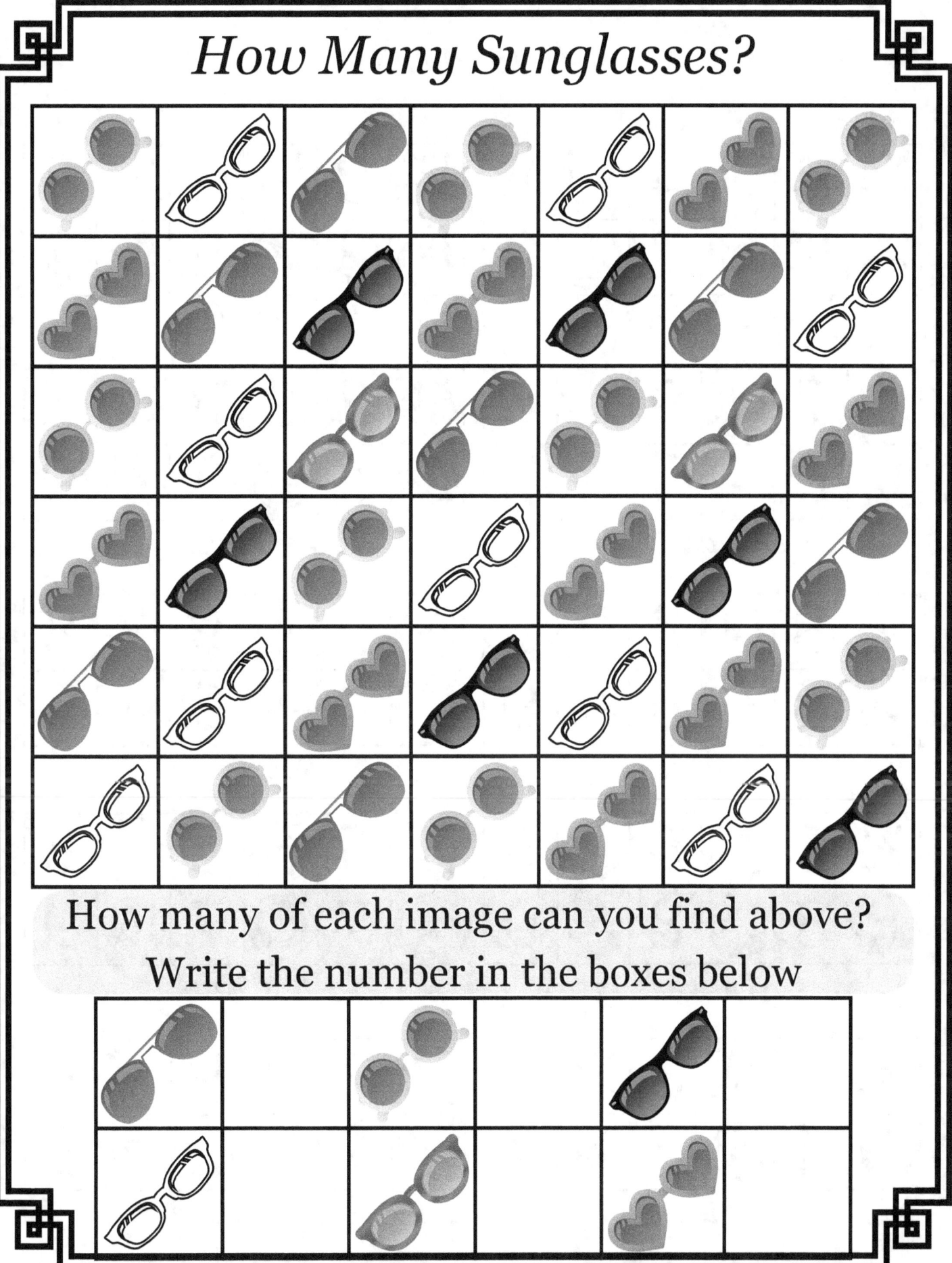

How many of each image can you find above?

Write the number in the boxes below

Answers

🧁	4	🧁	4	🧁	8
🧁	10	🧁	7	🧁	9

Cupcakes

🦉	8	🦉	4	🦉	8
🦉	8	🦉	5	🦉	9

Owls

🍂	7	🍁	9	🍃	6
🍃	8	🍁	5	🍃	7

Leaves

😀	8	👩	8	😟	5
😫	4	😊	8	😠	9

Faces

👠	8	👟	3	👢	8
🥾	8	🩴	6	👟	9

Shoes

🐵	9	🐵	9	🐵	8
🐵	4	🐵	9	🐵	3

Monkeys

🌻	5	🌼	6	🌸	6
🌹	8	🌷	8	🌺	9

Flowers

🔘	5	🔘	6	🔘	8
🔘	7	🔘	7	🔘	9

Buttons

🎩	9	🎩	8	🎩	7
🎩	4	🎩	7	🎩	7

Hats

🕶️	7	👓	9	🕶️	6
👓	9	🕶️	2	🕶️	9

Sunglasses

Crosswords

Fill in the puzzle
with the missing words
from the clues.

Crossword 1

Across

4 Birds of a _____ flock together.

6 Don't put all your eggs in one _____.

7 Every dark cloud has a silver _____.

9 Better safe than _____.

Down

1 Don't let the grass grow under your_____.

2 If you can't stand the heat, get out of the _____.

3 All's fair in love and _____.

5 A penny saved is a penny _____.

7 Actions speak _____ than words.

8 An apple a day keeps the doctor _____

Crossword 1

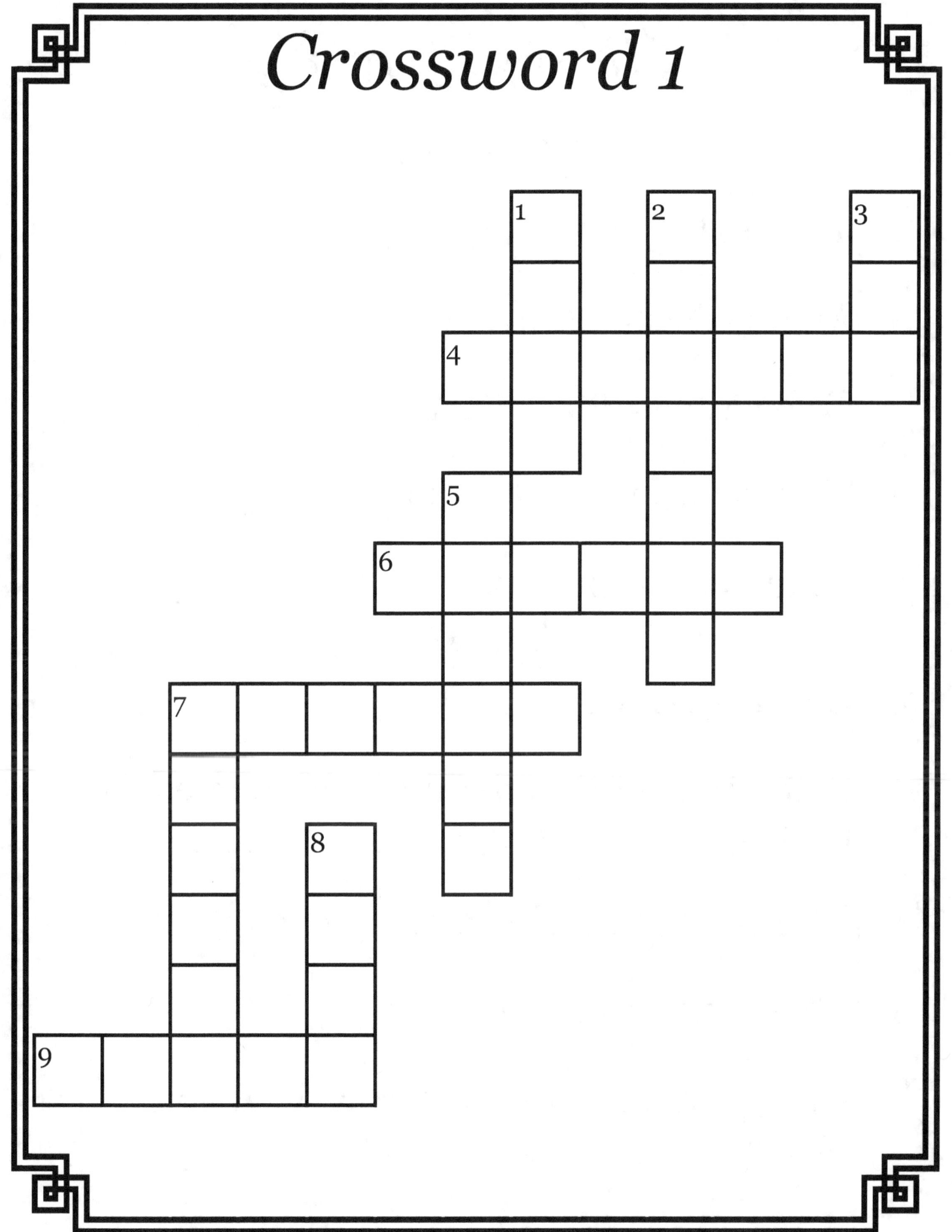

Crossword 2

Across

3 There's no place like _____ .

6 Money doesn't grow on _____ .

7 Two wrongs don't make a _____ .

9 Two heads are better than _____ .

10 Rome wasn't built in a _____ .

Down

1 Beggars can't be _____ .

2 Something old, something new, something borrowed, something _____ .

4 It's not worth crying over spilled_____ .

5 Three strikes and you're _____ .

8 Never put off until tomorrow what you can do _____ .

Crossword 2

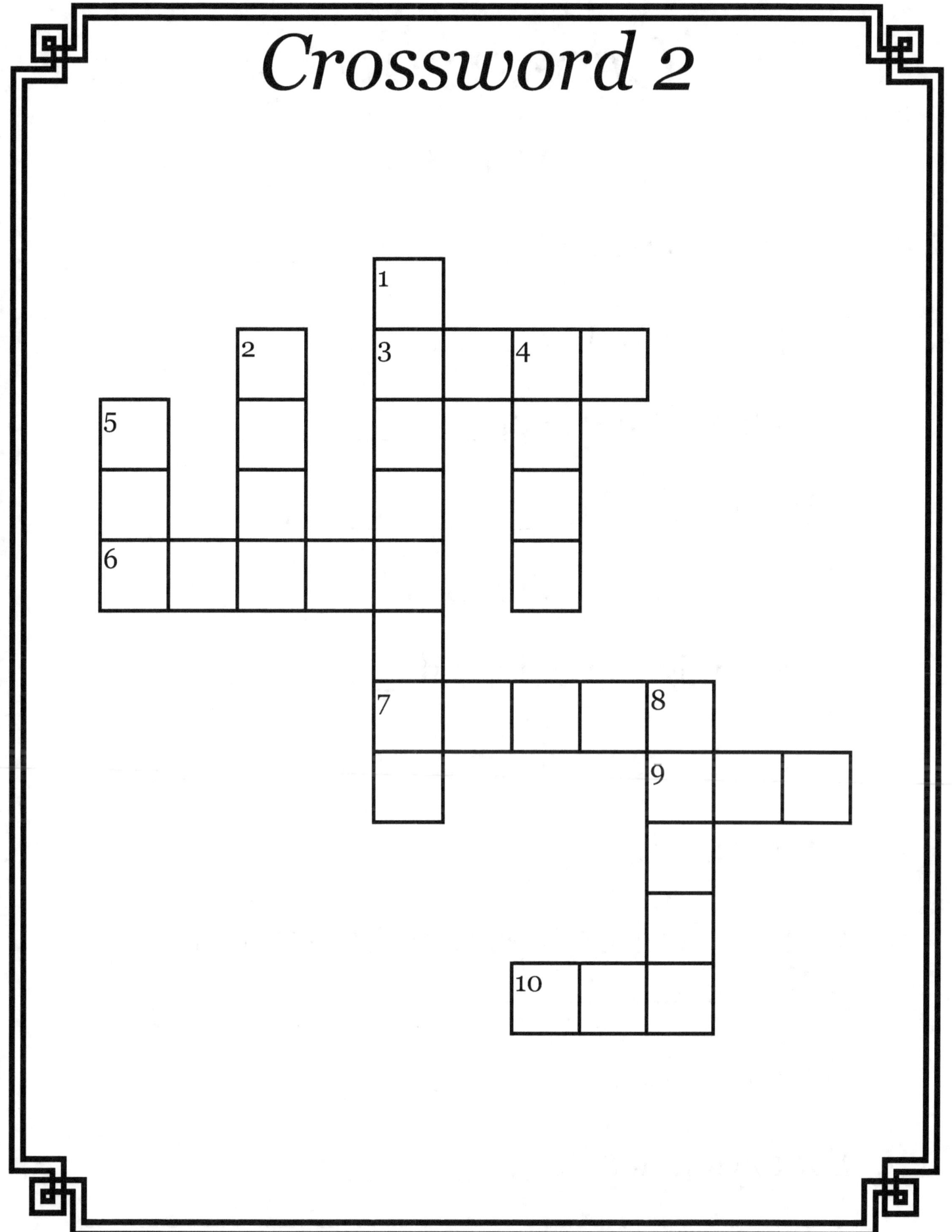

Crossword 3

Across

3 Put your best foot _____ .

5 They are a dime a _____ .

8 Laughter is the best _____ .

10 Like father, like _____ .

Down

1 Never judge a book by its_____ .

2 Where there is will there is a_____ .

4 A blessing in _____ .

6 You catch more flies with honey than with _____ .

7 When it rains it _____ .

9 Every dog has its _____ .

Crossword 3

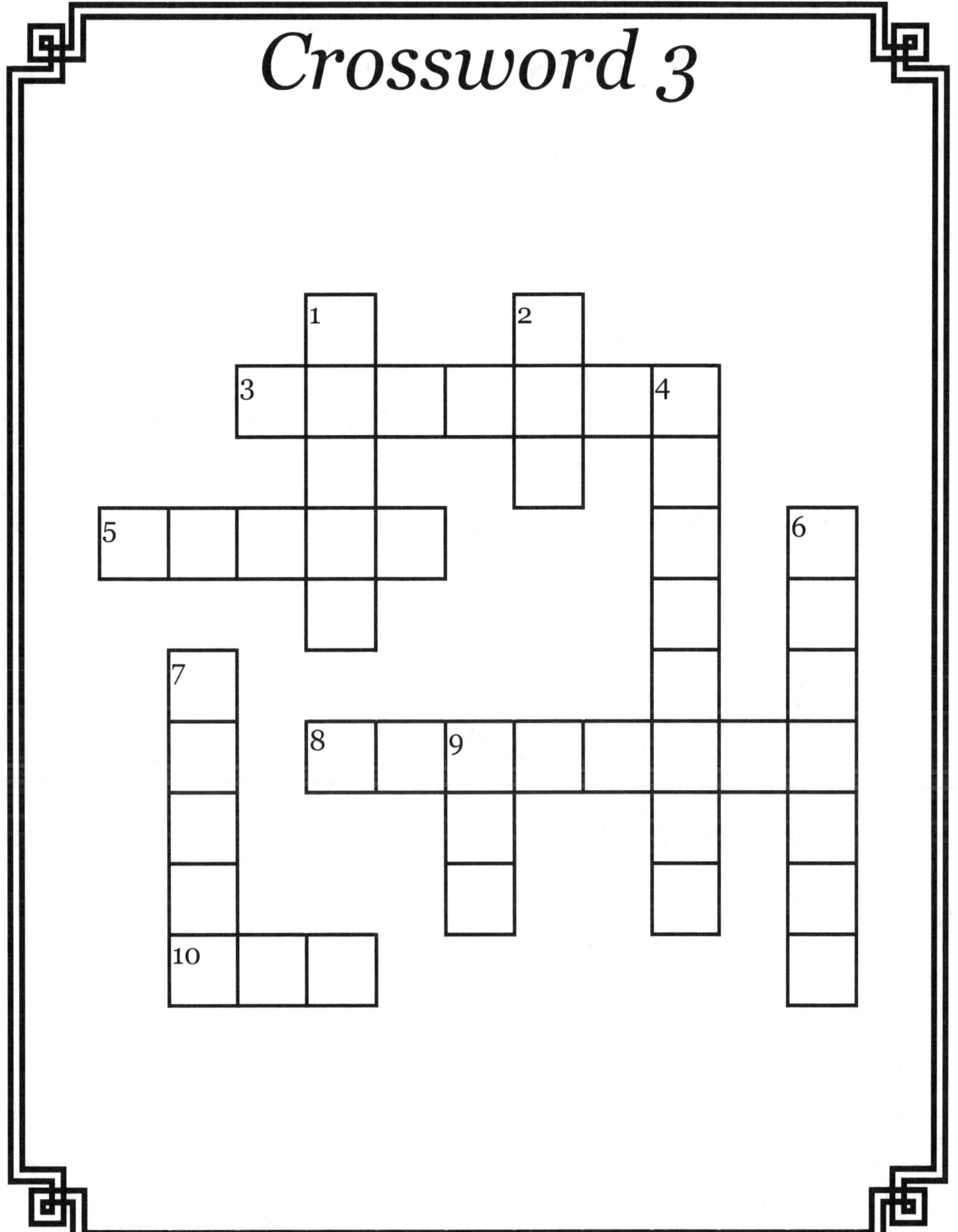

Crossword 4

Across

2 Caught between a rock and a hard_____ .

4 Adding insult to _____ .

5 _____ off more than you can chew.

7 Best of both _____ .

9 _____ around the bush.

Down

1 Doing something at the _____ of a hat.

3 Don't count your_____ before they hatch.

5 Bite the _____ .

6 Don't beat a dead _____ .

8 By the _____ of your teeth.

Crossword 4

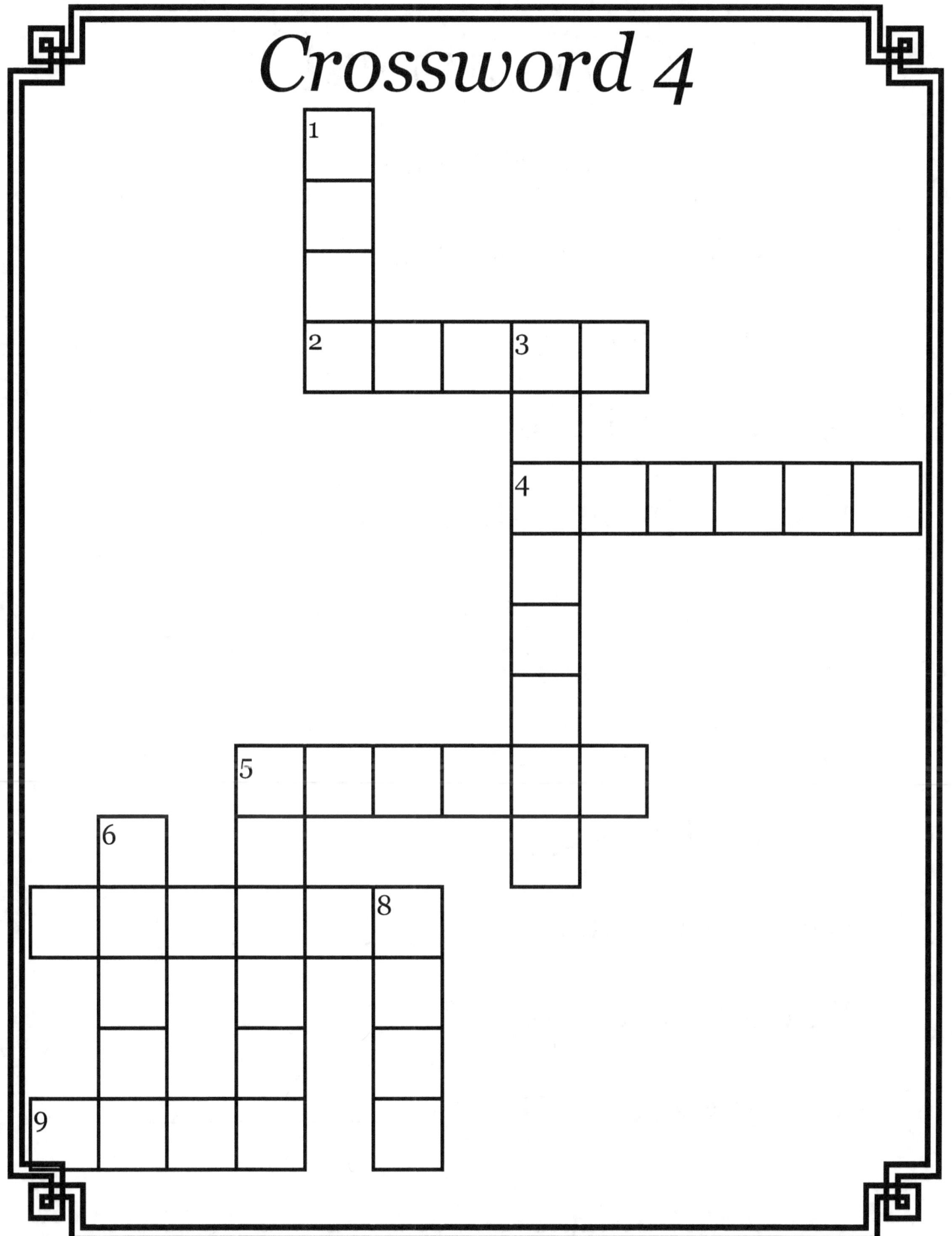

Crossword 5

Across

2 Giving the benefit of the _____ .

6 Feeling under the _____ .

7 Going on a wild goose _____ .

8 I heard it through the grape _____ .

9 _____ an arm and a leg.

Down

1 I'm fit as a _____ .

3 Getting the cold_____ .

4 Hitting the nail on the _____ .

6 Playing the devil's _____ .

7 Do a good job. Don't cut _____ .

Crossword 5

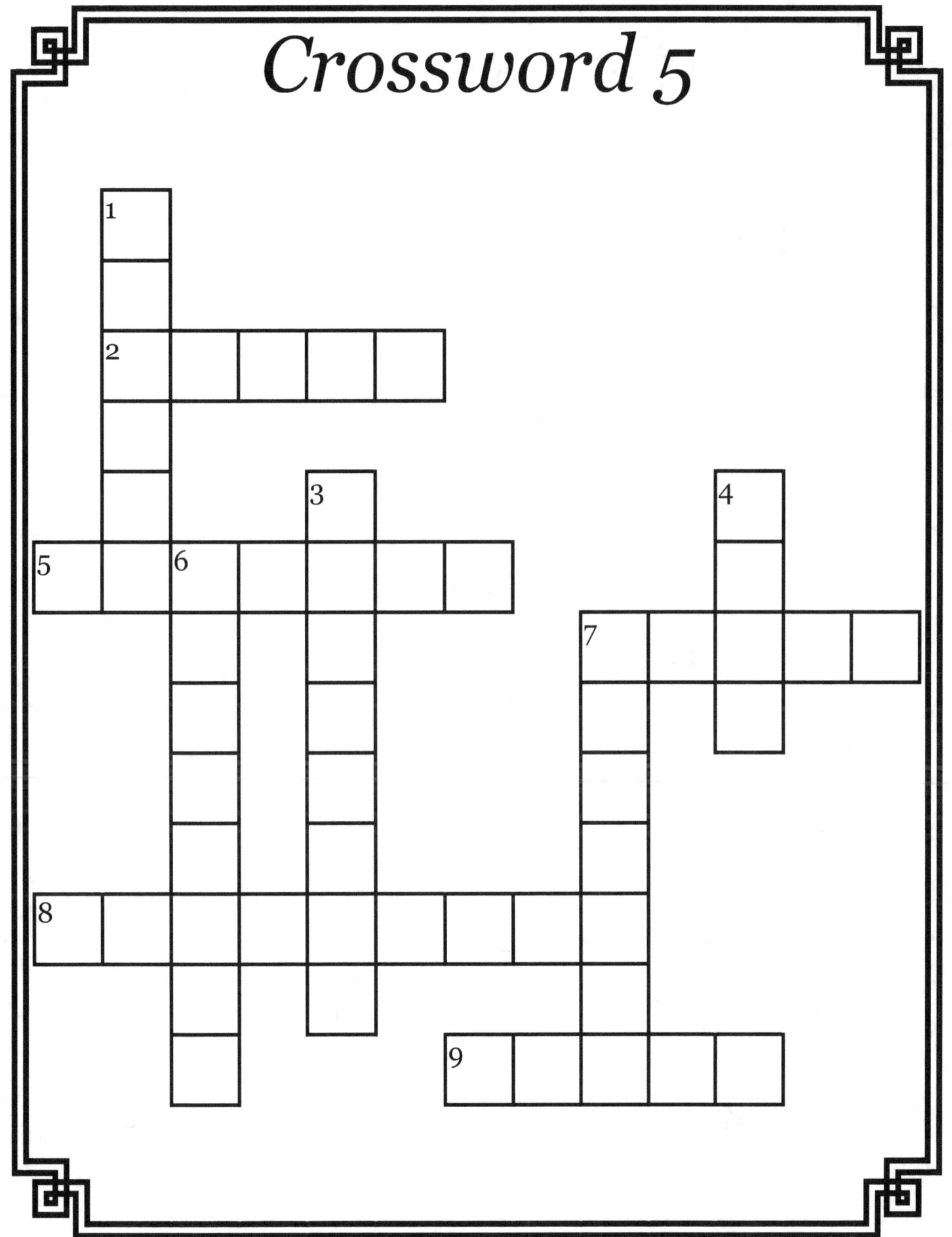

Crossword 6

Across

1 Killing two_____ with one stone.

6 Are you _____ my leg?

7 Stealing someone's _____ .

9 Once in a blue _____ .

Down

1 Letting the cat out of the _____ .

2 Heard it_____ from the horse's mouth.

3 Well, well, speak of the _____ .

4 No pain, no _____ .

5 Easy! Piece of _____ .

8 Letting someone off the _____ .

Crossword 6

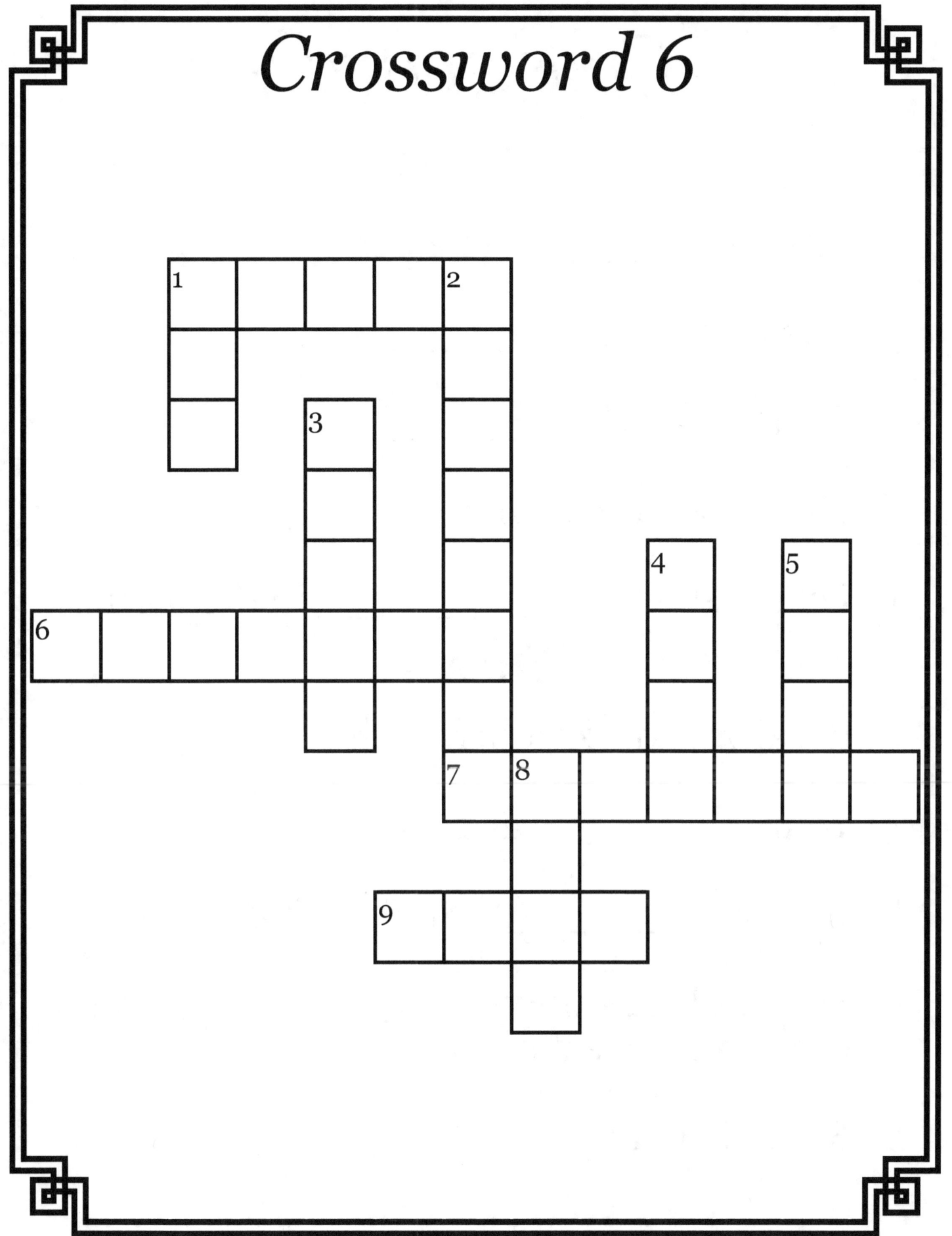

Crossword 7

Across

1 Like two_____ in a pod.

3 It takes two to _____ .

7 That was the last _____.

8 Having your head in the _____.

10 Let's addres the _____ in the room.

Down

1 It's always darkest before the _____ .

4 Your_____ is as good as.

5 Throw _____ to the wind.

6 You can lead a horse to_____, but
   you can't make it drink.

9 Better late than _____.

Crossword 7

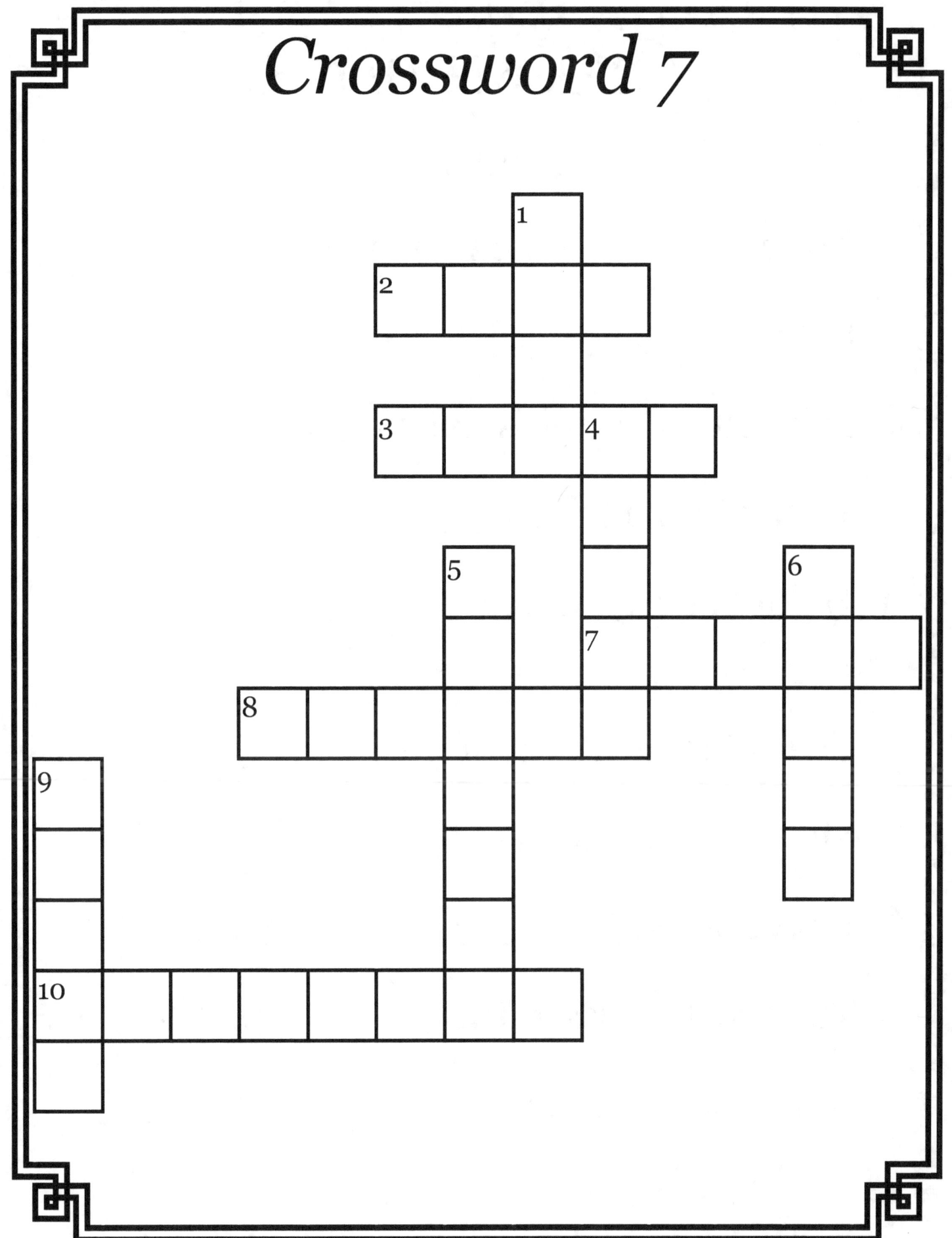

Crossword 8

Across

1 Time_____ when you're having fun.

4 So far so _____ .

5 It is difficult but it's not rocket_____.

7 We let him off the _____.

9 He did poorly. He cut _____ .

Down

2 I've got to get it out of my _____ .

3 She has to get her act_____ .

6 It will be ok. _____ in there.

8 They really missed the_____on that one.

10 I'm sleepy. I'm going to hit the_____.

Crossword 8

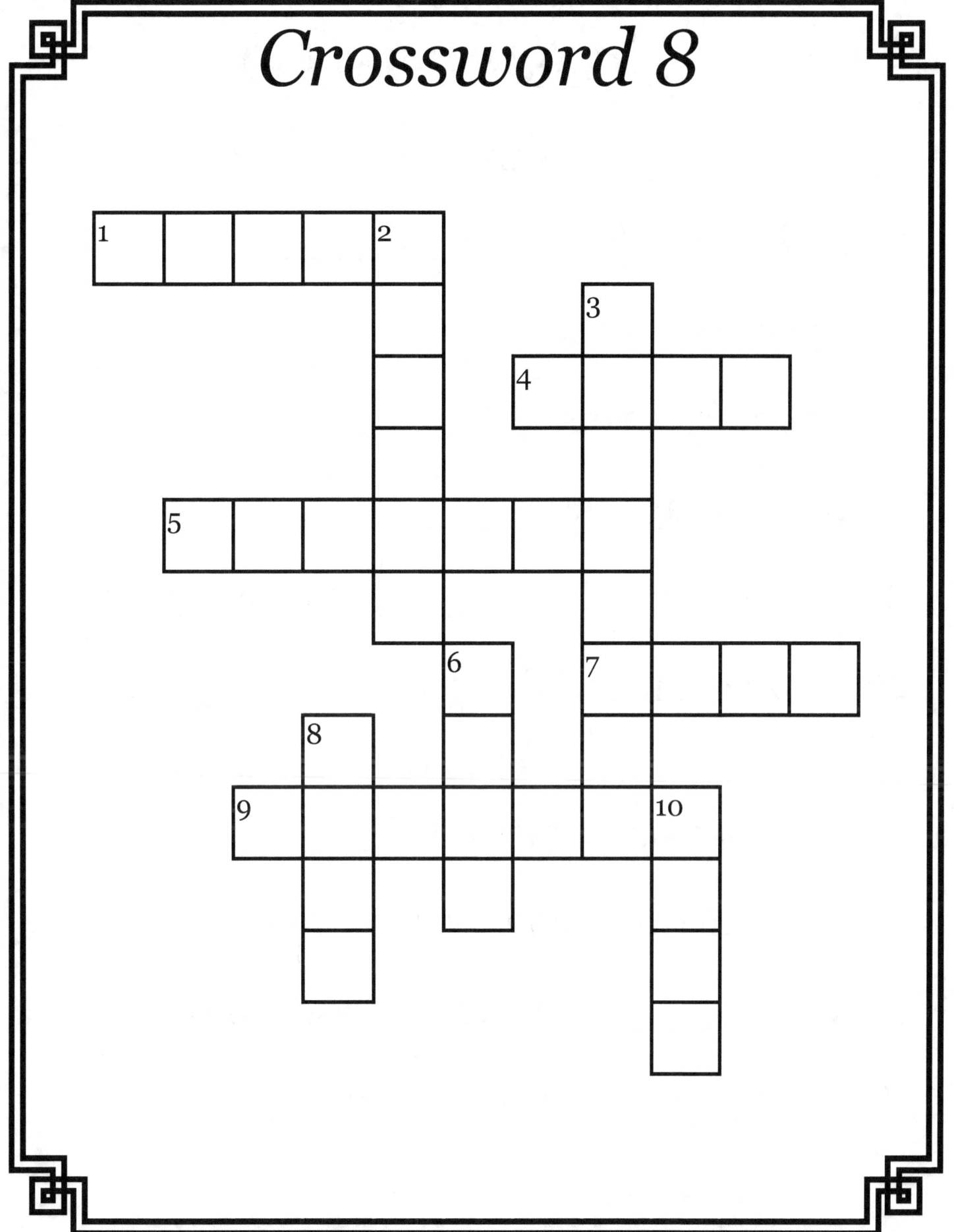

Crossword 9

Across

3 Barking up the wrong_____ .

4 To be bent out of_____ .

6 A penny for your_____.

8 You can say that _____.

9 We'll cross that _____ when we get to it.

10 We went on a wild goose_____.

Down

1 That only made matters _____ .

2 A bird in the hand is worth two in the_____ .

5 A _____ is worth 1000 words.

7 You can't compare apples to_____.

Crossword 9

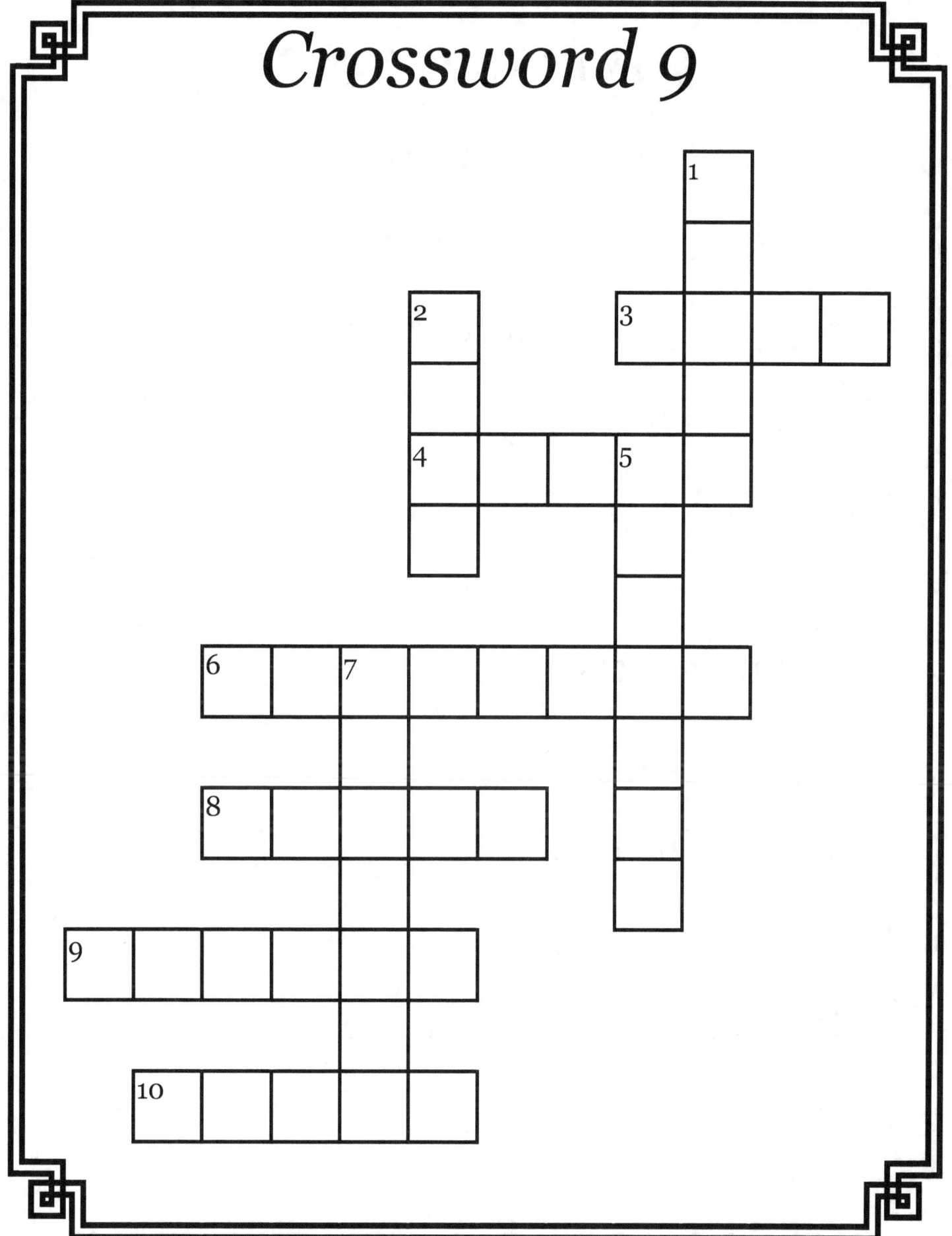

Crossword 10

Across

3 I have_____ fish to fry.

6 It_____ one to know one.

7 Oh well. Live and_____.

8 Slow and steady wins the _____.

Down

1 It's raining cats and _____ .

2 Rain on someone's _____ .

3 He's a chip off the old _____ .

4 Save it for a _____ day.

5 She really hit the nail on the _____ .

7 Look before you _____ .

Crossword 10

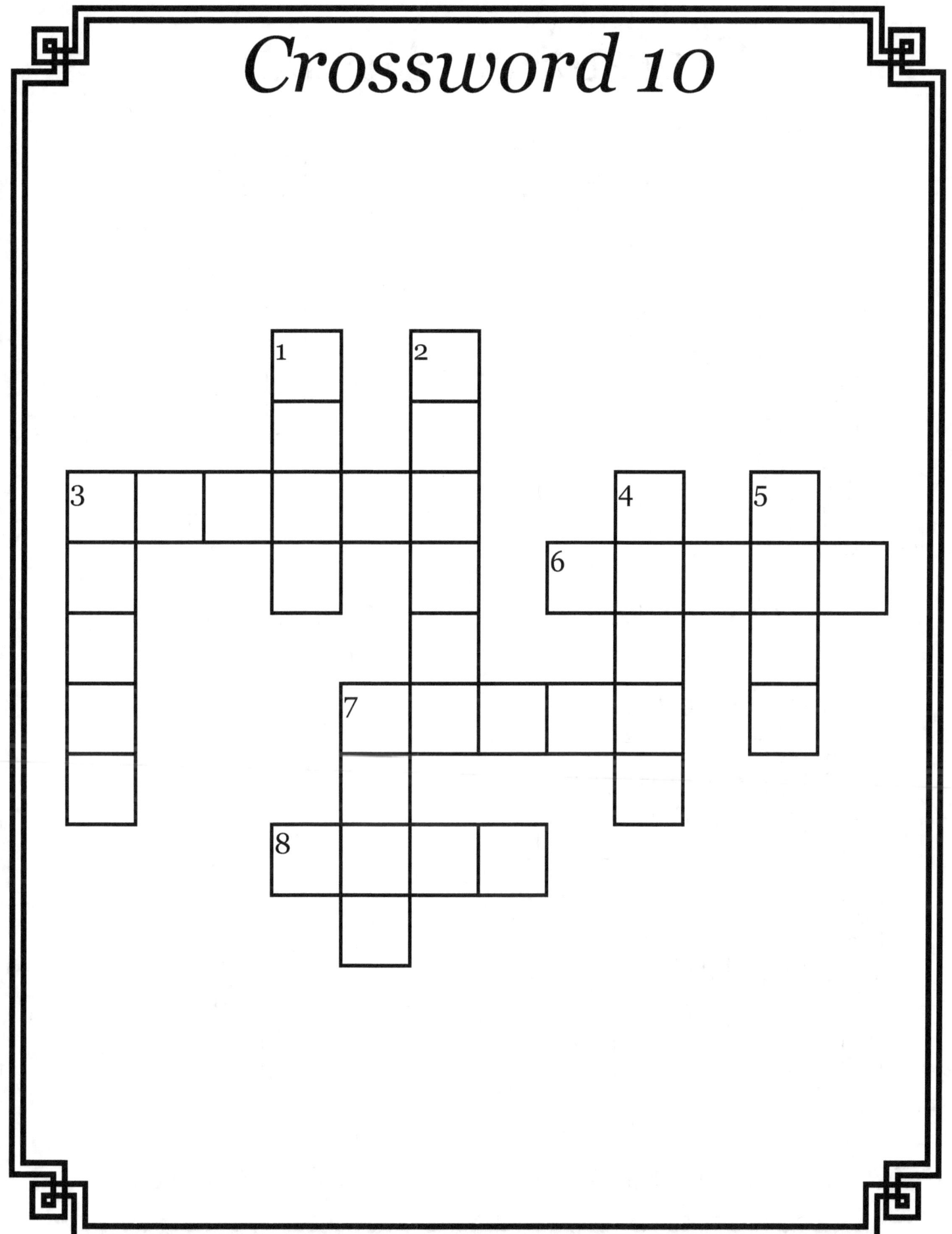

Crossword Answers

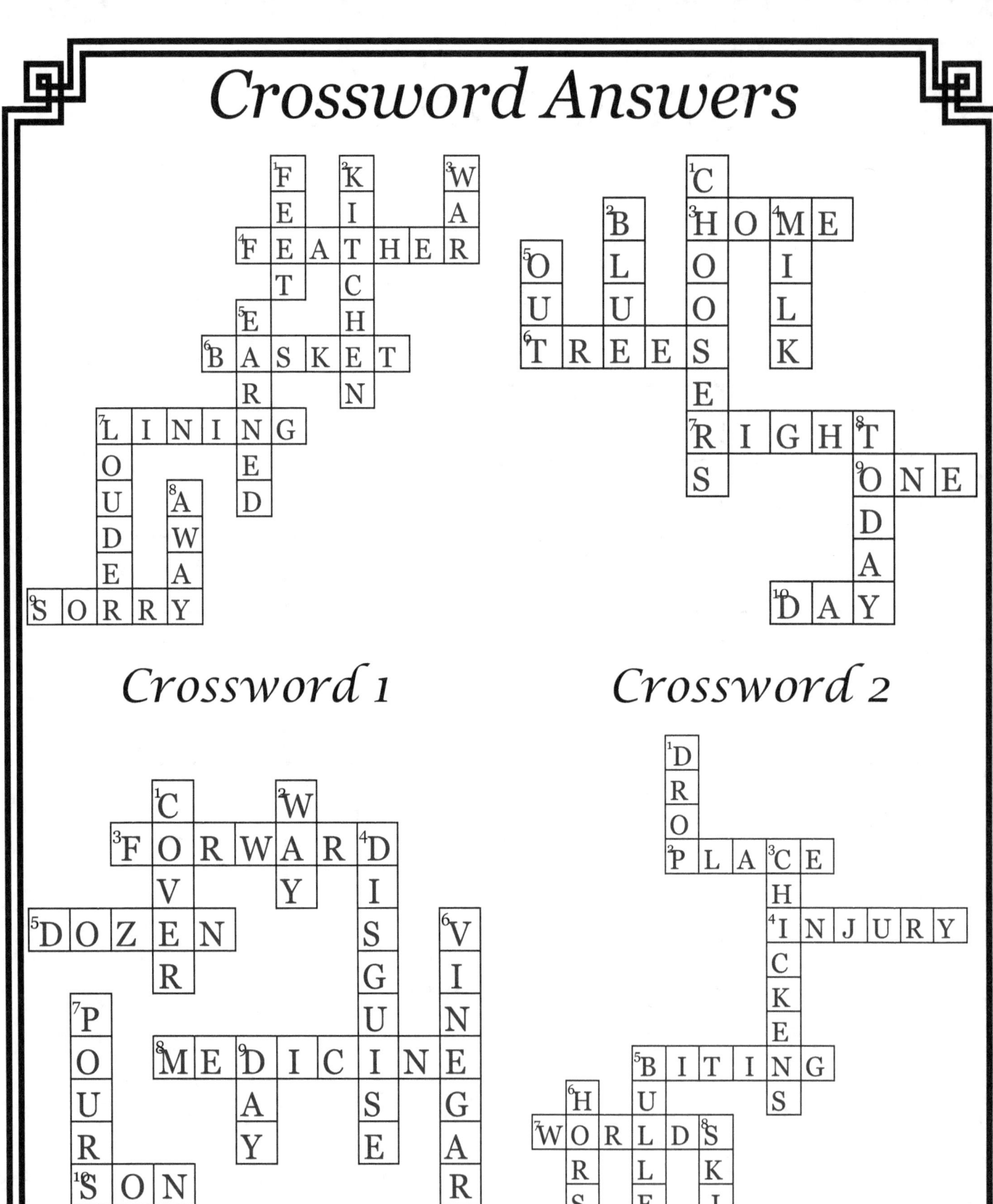

Crossword 1

Crossword 2

Crossword 3

Crossword 4

Crossword Answers

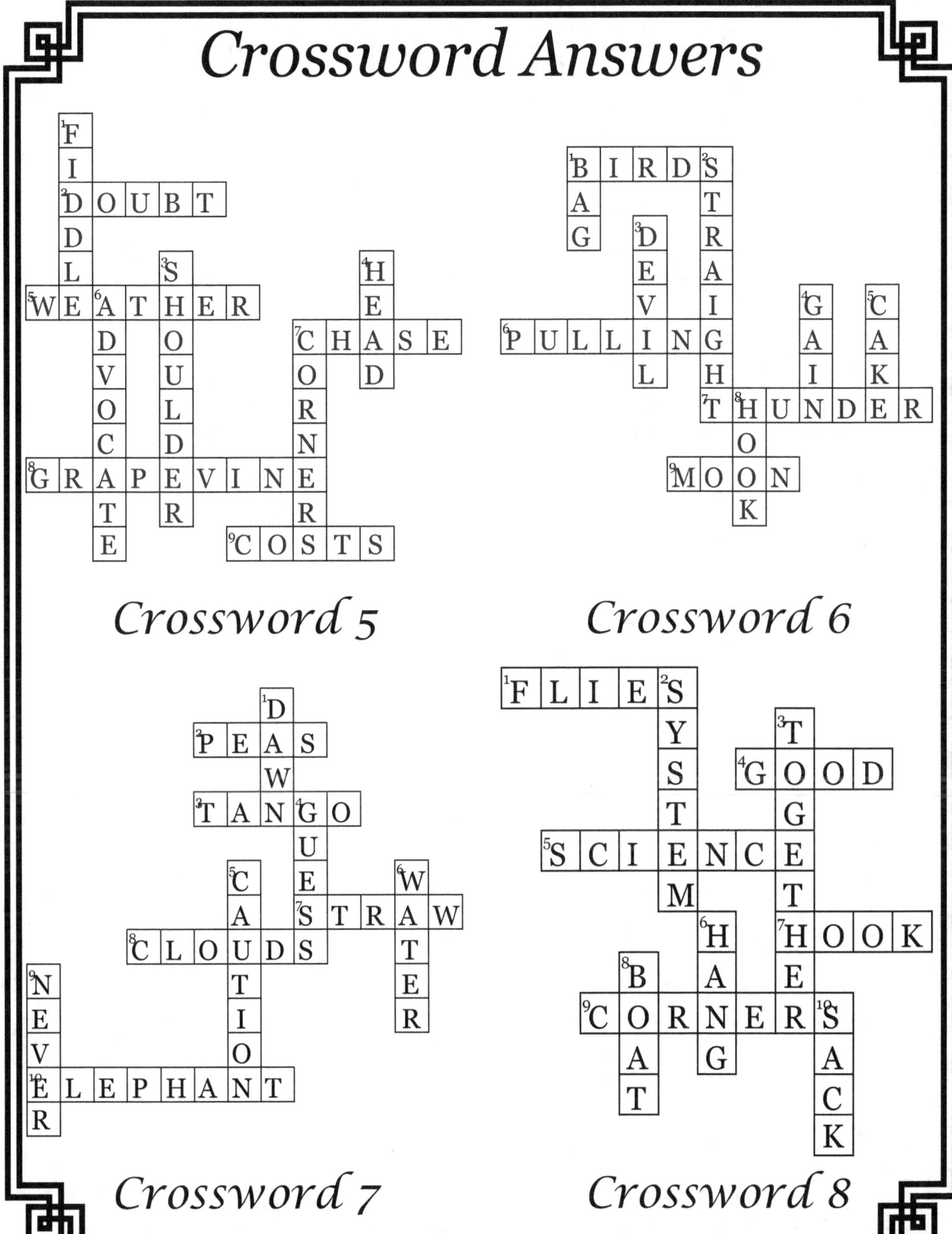

Crossword 5

F
I
D
D
DOUBT
L
E S
WEATHER   H
D O E
V U C **CHASE**   A
O L O D
C D R
A E N
GRAPEVINE R
T E
E R
S
COSTS

Crossword 6

BIRDS   S
A T
G R
D A
E I G C
V G A A
PULLING H A K
L T **THUNDER**
O
MOON K

Crossword 7

D
PEAS
A
W
TANGO
U
C E
CAUTION   W
A **STRAW** A
CLOUDS T
N A E
E T R
V I
E **ELEPHANT**
R

Crossword 8

FLIES   S
Y T
S **GOOD**
T O
SCIENCE G
M E
H T
B A **HOOK**
CORNER   S
O G A
A C
T K

Crossword Answers

Crossword 9

```
              ¹W
               O
               R
    ²B    ³T  R  E  E
     U        S
    ⁴S  H  A  ⁵P  E
     H        I
              C
    ⁶T  H  ⁷O  U  G  H  T  S
     A    R   C
    ⁸A  G  A  ⁷I  N  T
     N        U
    ⁹B  R  I  D  G  E  R
              E
    ¹⁰C  H  A  S  E
```

Crossword 10

```
           ¹D        ²P
            O         A
    ³B  I  G  G  E  R  A       ⁴R        ⁵H
     L      S         A    ⁶T  A  K  E  S
     O                D     E  A  R  N  Y  A
     C          ⁷L  E  A  R  N  Y     A  D
     K           E        E     N
              ⁸R  A  C  E          Y
                 P
```

Mazes

Find the path from
start to finish.

Maze 1

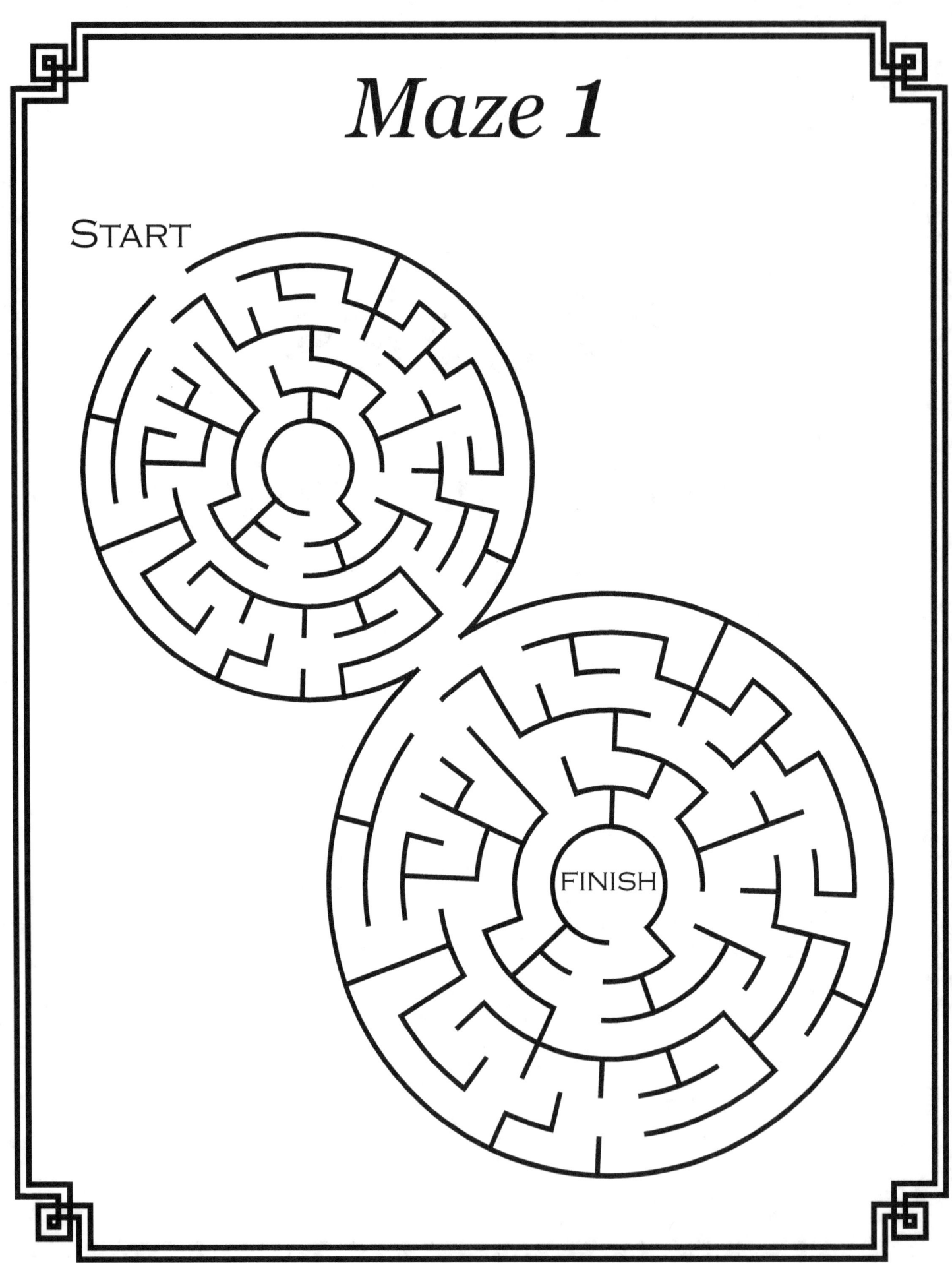

START

FINISH

Maze 2

START

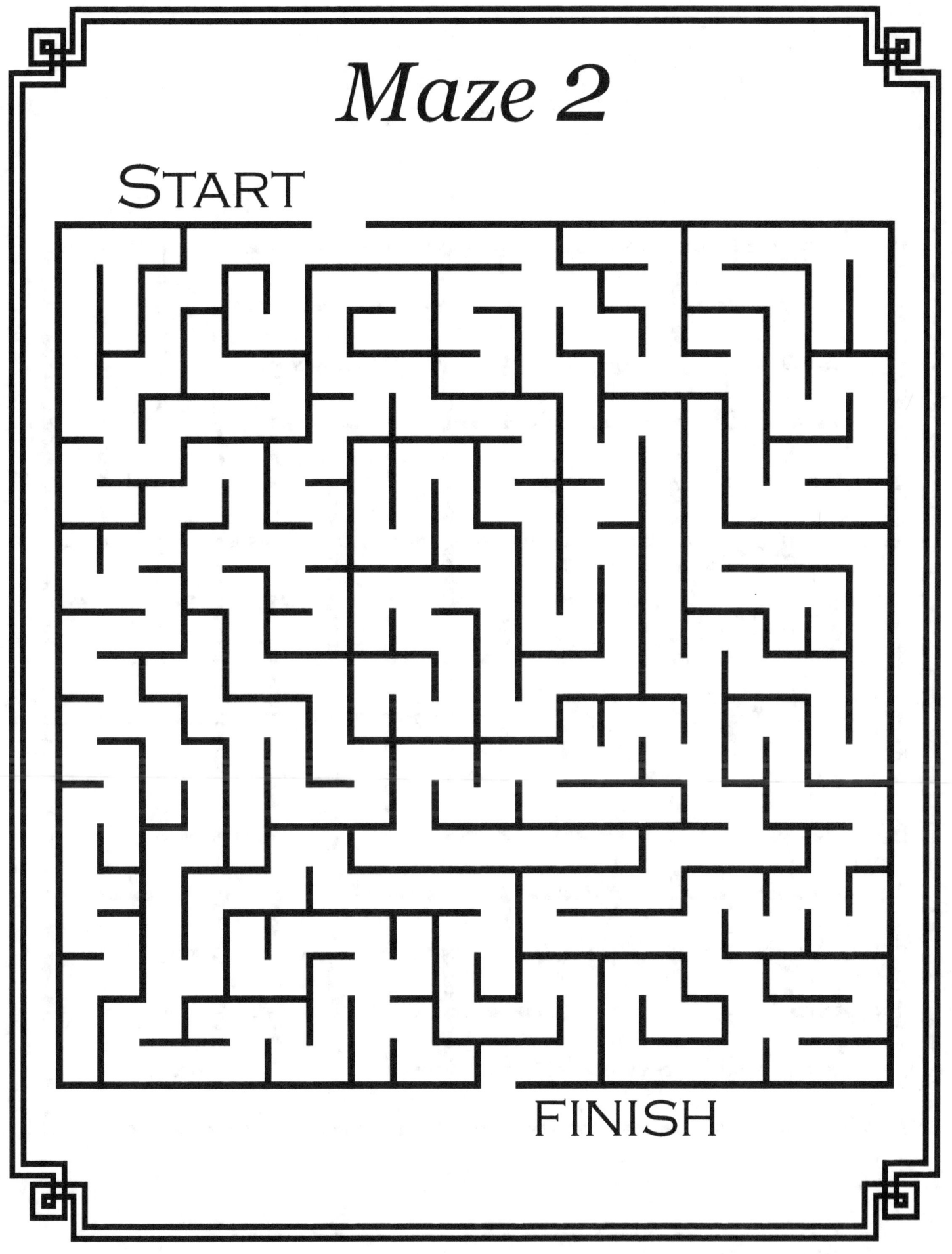

FINISH

Maze 3

START

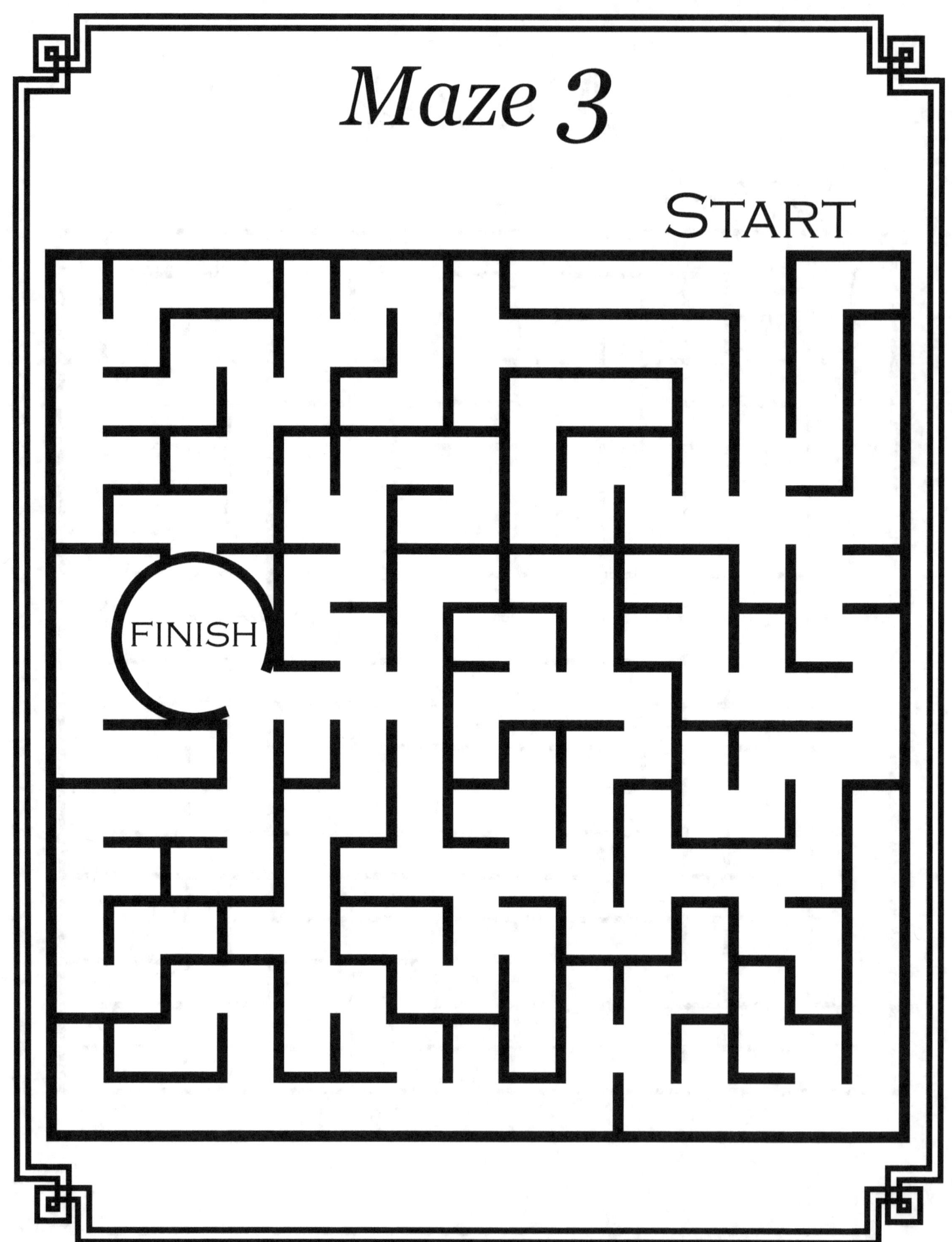

FINISH

Maze 4

Start

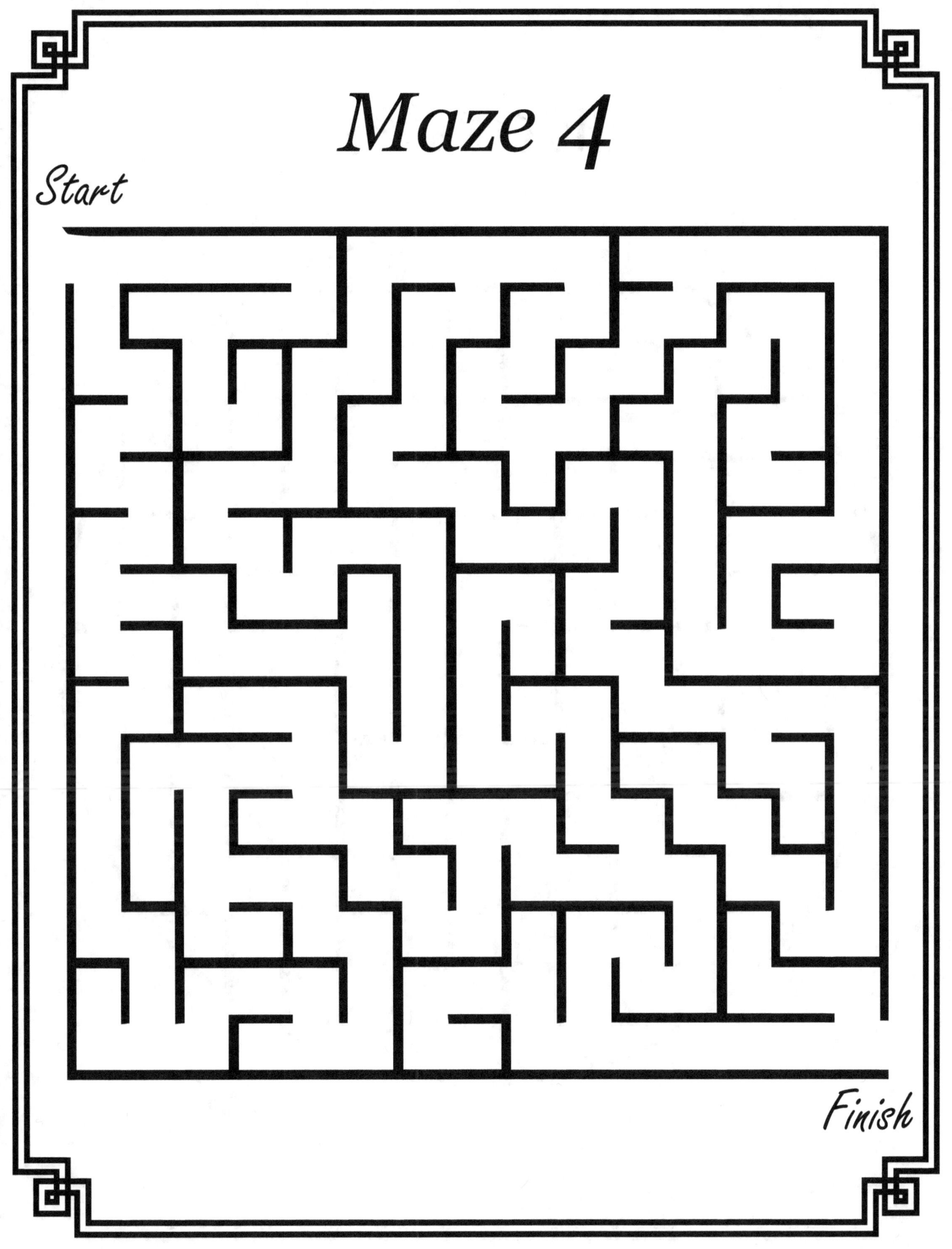

Finish

Maze 5

Start

Finish

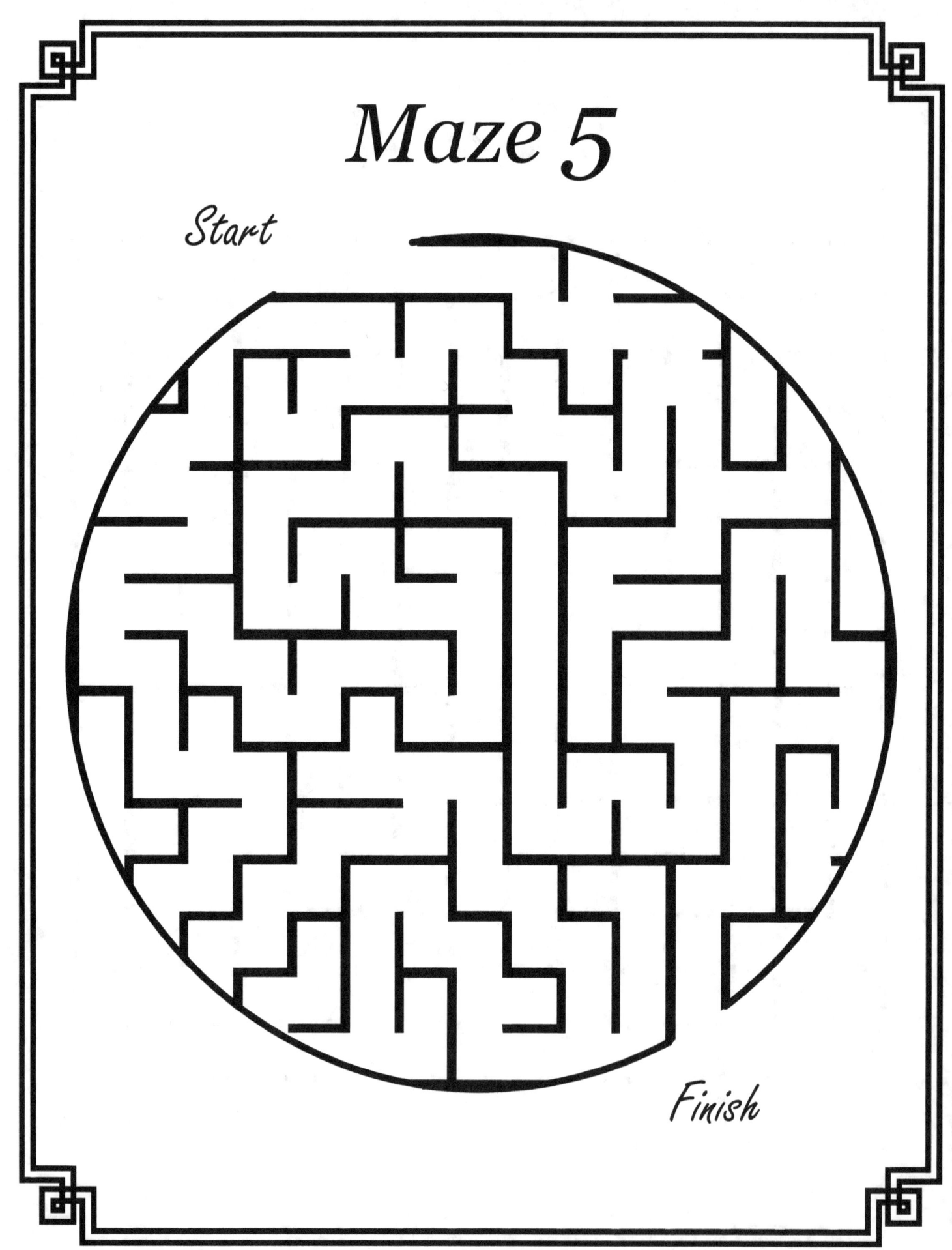

Maze 6

Start

Finish

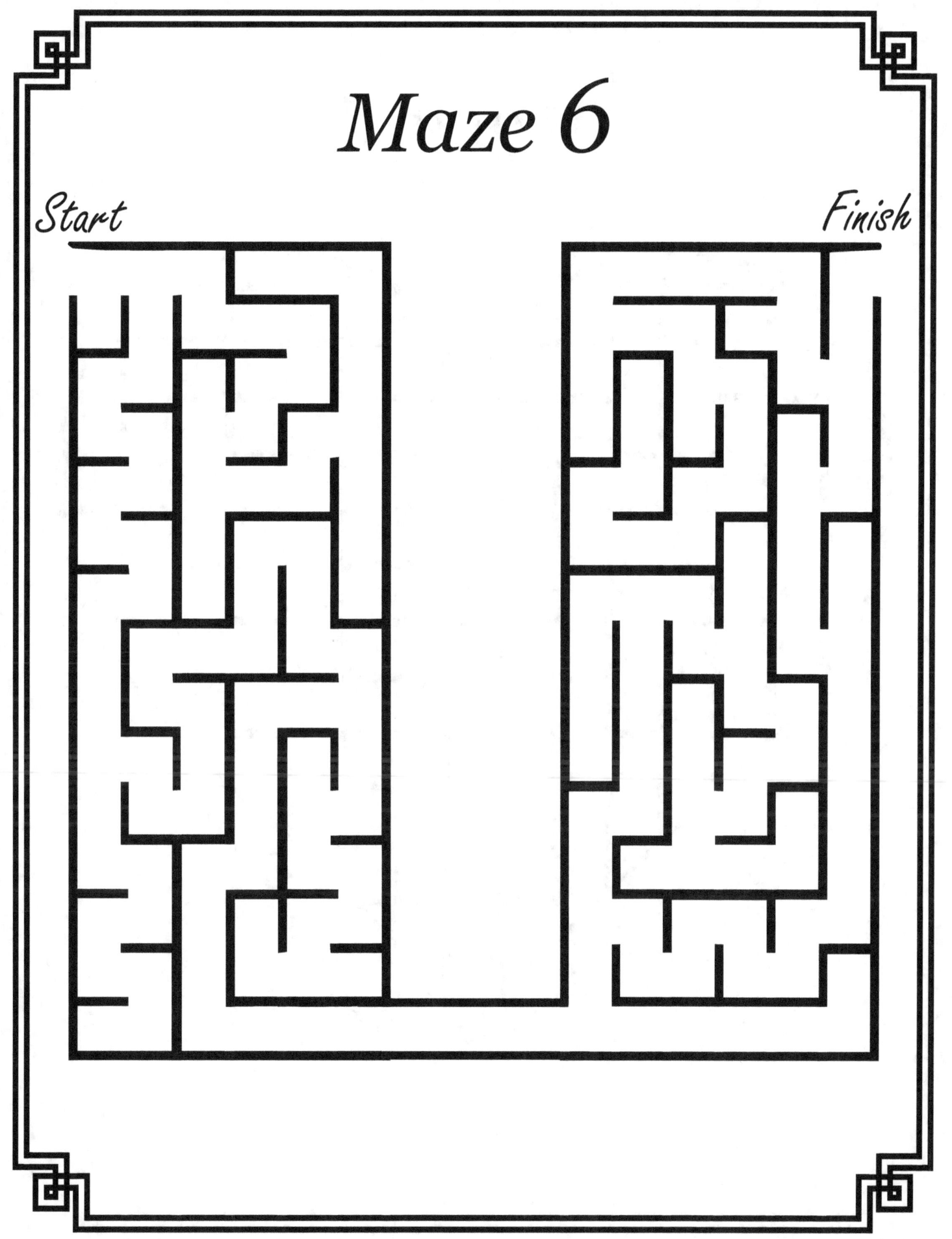

Maze 7

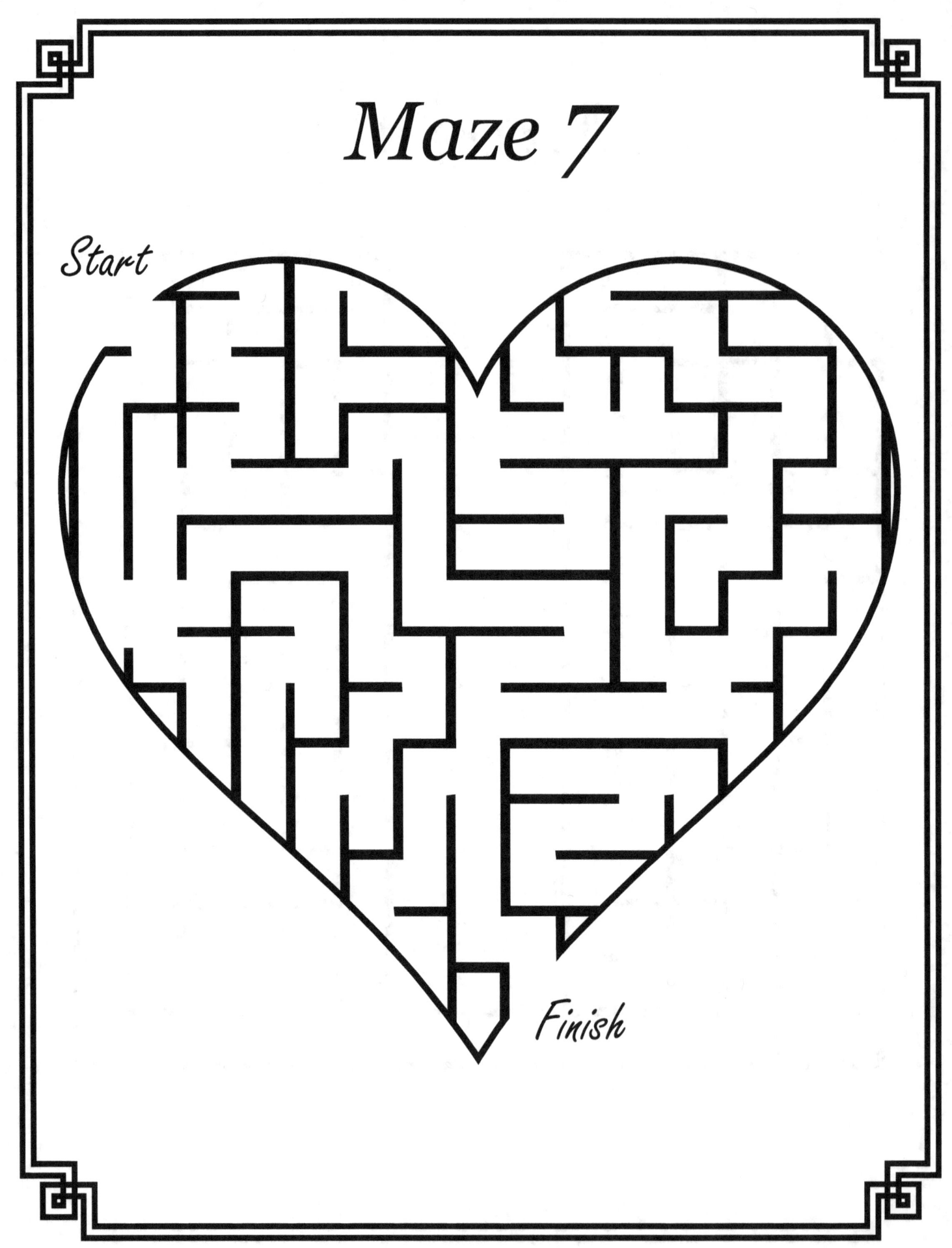

Maze 8

Start

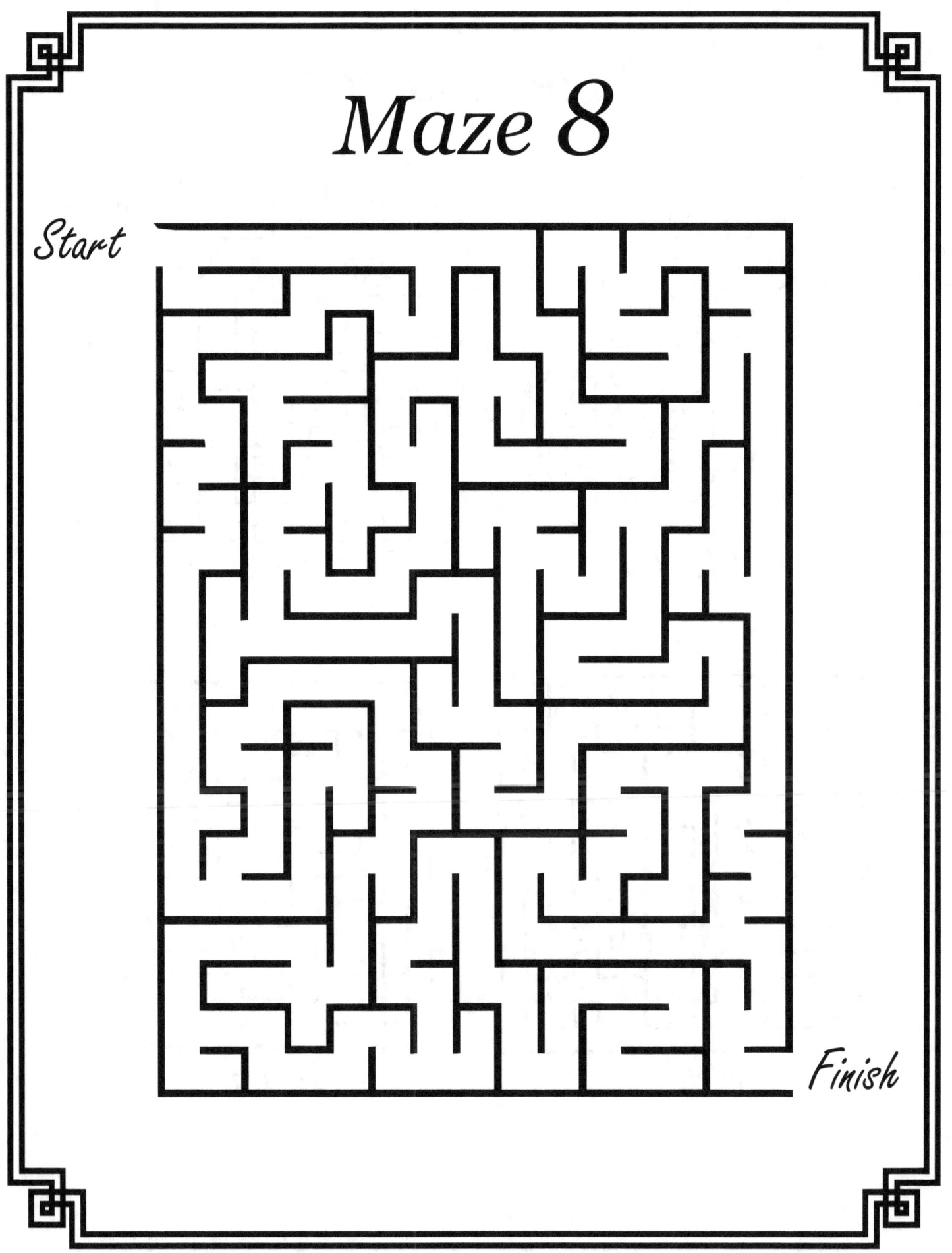

Finish

Maze Answers

Maze 1

Maze 2

Maze 3

Maze 4

Maze Answers

Maze 5

Maze 6

Maze 7

Maze 8

Memory Challenge!

Remember the list of unrelated words. Flip the page and write as many of the words as you can.

Remember these words:

1. TOOTHBRUSH
2. APPLE
3. CHAIR
4. RHYME
5. VASE
6. PURPLE
7. TANK
8. CANNON
9. REQUEST
10. COMMUNICATE
11. EXCLUSIVE
12. WIRY

Write the words from the last page

1. _____

2. _____

3. _____

4. _____

5. _____

6. _____

7. _____

8. _____

9. _____

10. _____

11. _____

12. _____

Flip back to check your answers.

Remember these words:

1. TAP
2. TROUSERS
3. TESTY
4. WASH
5. TIRE
6. DESIRE
7. HEAT
8. FETCH
9. BEAR
10. FLAP
11. SAME
12. MELLOW

Write the words from the last page

1. _____
2. _____
3. _____
4. _____
5. _____
6. _____
7. _____
8. _____
9. _____
10. _____
11. _____
12. _____

Flip back to check your answers.

Remember these words:

1. COLOR
2. UNKNOWN
3. HOLIDAY
4. DIFFICULT
5. TIP
6. LITERATE
7. SHUT
8. REST
9. AUTHORITY
10. AIRPORT
11. COUGH
12. VALUABLE

Write the words from the last page

1. _____
2. _____
3. _____
4. _____
5. _____
6. _____
7. _____
8. _____
9. _____
10. _____
11. _____
12. _____

Flip back to check your answers.

Remember these words:

1. DEBONAIR
2. AHEAD
3. ASH
4. WONDER
5. THEORY
6. CENT
7. ROOM
8. PLAIN
9. RESTFULL
10. ORANGE
11. NUMBER
12. ELITE

Write the words from the last page

1. _____
2. _____
3. _____
4. _____
5. _____
6. _____
7. _____
8. _____
9. _____
10. _____
11. _____
12. _____

Flip back to check your answers.

Remember these words:

1. CHANGE
2. KNOCK
3. BOAT
4. COMPANY
5. BUTTON
6. ALLEGED
7. CELEBRATE
8. ARMY
9. ALOOF
10. FISH
11. CRABBY
12. AROMA

Write the words from the last page

1. _____
2. _____
3. _____
4. _____
5. _____
6. _____
7. _____
8. _____
9. _____
10. _____
11. _____
12. _____

Flip back to check your answers.

Remember these words:

1. PUZZLING
2. FIT
3. KNOTTY
4. DESSERT
5. OVERFLOW
6. ANALYSIS
7. GRANDIOSE
8. LACE
9. ATTEMPT
10. THAW
11. SLIP
12. TESTED

Write the words from the last page

1. _____

2. _____

3. _____

4. _____

5. _____

6. _____

7. _____

8. _____

9. _____

10. _____

11. _____

12. _____

Flip back to check your answers.

Remember these words:

1. KNOWING
2. OCCUR
3. ENDLESS
4. CIRCLE
5. SCATTER
6. AWARE
7. RAGGED
8. PICTURE
9. SPELL
10. INTELLIGENT
11. TELLING
12. OPPOSITE

Write the words from the last page

1. _____
2. _____
3. _____
4. _____
5. _____
6. _____
7. _____
8. _____
9. _____
10. _____
11. _____
12. _____

Flip back to check your answers.

Remember these words:

1. HOP
2. SUCCINCT
3. SQUEEK
4. TANK
5. LIGHTEN
6. WELL
7. TIDY
8. FLOW
9. SMILE
10. DESTROY
11. EARLY
12. BROOM

Write the words from the last page

1. _____
2. _____
3. _____
4. _____
5. _____
6. _____
7. _____
8. _____
9. _____
10. _____
11. _____
12. _____

Flip back to check your answers.

Remember these words:

1. WACKY
2. TIGHT
3. DOMINATE
4. FILE
5. MARK
6. FIVE
7. LICENSE
8. STANDING
9. INVITE
10. FLAVOR
11. FROG
12. SOMBER

Write the words from the last page

1. _____
2. _____
3. _____
4. _____
5. _____
6. _____
7. _____
8. _____
9. _____
10. _____
11. _____
12. _____
13. _____
14. _____

Flip back to check your answers.

Remember these words:

1. COORDINATE
2. NEEDED
3. SUSPEND
4. PRICEY
5. GRANDMOM
6. THIN
7. EXCHANGE
8. ROOMY
9. TEACHING
10. RAILWAY
11. SMOOTH
12. FINGER
13. TASTEFUL
14. LUNCHROOM

Write the words from the last page

1. _____

2. _____

3. _____

4. _____

5. _____

6. _____

7. _____

8. _____

9. _____

10. _____

11. _____

12. _____

13. _____

14. _____

Flip back to check your answers.

Remember these words:

1. CLIP
2. SHOE
3. ADVENTURE
4. PANCAKE
5. START
6. UNDERWEAR
7. RABBITS
8. GOVERNMENT
9. MEND
10. RESCUE
11. TRY
12. GEESE
13. WEALTHY
14. RINGS

Write the words from the last page

1. _____

2. _____

3. _____

4. _____

5. _____

6. _____

7. _____

8. _____

9. _____

10. _____

11. _____

12. _____

13. _____

14. _____

Flip back to check your answers.

Please leave a review!

⭐ ⭐ ⭐ ⭐ ⭐